Soul Medicine

A Physician's Reflections
on Life, Love, Death and Healing

Judith Boice, N.D., L.Ac., FABNO

Soul Medicine:

*A Physician's Reflections
on Life, Love, Death and Healing*

Copyright © 2016 by Judith Boice,

Edited by Phyllis Ring
Book design by Jeremy Berg
Cover art by Missy Rogers
Interior Images:
Winter scene: by Paul/Shutterstock.com
White flowers: Anna Omelchenko/Shutterstock.com
Bird: sysasya/Shutterstock.com
Forest with mist: siloto/Shutterstock.com

Published by Lorian Press
6592 Peninsula Dr.
Traverse City, MI 49686

ISBN-13: 978-0-936878-83-6

Boice, Judith
*Soul Medicine: A Physician's Reflections on Life, Love, Death
and Healing/*Judith Boice

Library of Congress Control Number: 2016944295

First Edition July 2016

Printed in the United States of America

0 9 8 7 6 5 4 3 2 1

www.lorian.org

Dedication

To Kathleen Welsh Luiten and the Masters, the Ancient Ones, for your unwavering love, wisdom and support.

TABLE OF CONTENTS

SUMMER

AUTUMN

Acknowledgments

I am grateful for all the fellow travelers who have shared their journeys with me. Your stories have enriched my life beyond measure. May this book provide a loving spoonful in return.

Thank you to the crew at KVNF in Paonia, Colorado – especially Jeff Reynolds, Sally Kane and all of the DJs – for your support in creating and producing "The Mystic's Almanac" radio show, the inspiration for the essays in this book.

Many thanks to Phyllis Ring for her expert editing eye.

A deep bow of gratitude to David Spangler, Jeremy Berg and Lorian Press for your support in birthing these stories into the wider world.

Many thanks to Missy Rogers for applying her fine eye and even finer heart in creating the cover and interior images.

Special thanks to my sons, Vincent and Sebastian, for providing endless grist for smoothing every rough edge I thought I had long since abandoned (and for creating a few new ones . . . .) I love you beyond measure.

"Bare Bones Landscape" first appeared in 2009©, and is reprinted with permission from Bereavement Publications, Inc., Living With Loss™ Magazine.

Praise for Soul Medicine

Poetic . . . haunting, and much of it fascinating and insightful.

Dr. Rick Kirschner, *Dealing with People You Can't Stand*

Judith's book is the essence of story-telling as medicine. Each vignette evokes in us something that calls out to be healed. The reader will be carried down the stream of their own past with the assurance that they are not alone. Her vulnerable and open-hearted narrative reminds us what it is to be human and to aspire towards wholeness. I want to read it slowly...again and again.

Dr. Yvonne Farrell, DAOM, *Psycho-Emotional Pain and the Eight Extraordinary Vessels*

This book is a kaleidoscope of personal reflections, thoughtful musings and memories, and social commentaries from a doctor's life filled with meaning and intention. It's often touching, at times quirky, and consistently light-hearted and filled with sacred good will.

Vicki Noble, Co-creator of Motherpeace, author of *Shakti Woman* and *The Double Goddess*

With Soul Medicine, my Judith (we worked together, fellow physicians) creates a calm harbor in the pandemonium of daily life. She shares with us the wonderment, mystery, and awe of her vision of our earth as well as the spirit/spiritual world that surrounds us, constantly, silently begging for recognition with signs and premonitions, and grace. This collection of essays, metaphorically separated into the seasons of the year, and of life, will bring you joy.

G. L. River, MD, FACP, Medical Oncologist, Tulsa, OK

Dr. Judith Boice writes with the heart of a philosopher and the voice of a poet. Every chapter is like a bite of a delicious meal, to be savored. Take your time and let her words nourish you.

Louise Edwards, ND, Naturopathic Physician, Faculty at National University of Health Sciences

FOREWORD

Oh, golly! I began to read these essays as a task to which I had agreed, somewhat reluctantly. My old student, Judith Boice, now Dr. Boice, asked me to write a forward for her latest book. Her invitation had come just before the New Year's holiday weekend. I could make the time to do this favor for an old student, but I had other things to write. I planned to use the long weekend to rest from a difficult year. But the time came to open the book, and I began to read.

Two hours later I realized that I had been drawn into the delightful mind of Judith, a process she describes in the essay, "The Book Slut." I could not stop reading. This was no task. This was a feast of unexpected delicacies, foreign but delightful flavors, spices I had not known. I had discovered an alley in an unfamiliar city that led to explorations I had not sought but that I could not resist. I found myself chuckling as I read "Bare Bones Landscape," and deeply struck by a poignant moment in the chapter, "Sonja Bullaty." The theme of family is strong in Judith's work, and very feminine: see "River of Ancestors," "From the Inside Out," or "No Regrets." As I read, I can smell the soil of her gardening, and remember being inside the hollow of a massive old tree, in my case a cedar, not an oak. She writes as an American, but with an international perspective. She has walked elsewhere, and we feel it in these pages, as we read of holding hands with children in the Australian desert in "Inner and Outer Technology." I remembered some of my own explorations as a young man, of the different cultures I had encountered, and the paths that led me to my career in our tiny profession, a hidden medicine.

I write as a professor of medicine and not of literature. I cannot comment upon her comparison to other writers, to Thoreau or Wendell Berry, or those sorts of things. I'm a novice at this. But I was continually struck by the simple, well-crafted statements, like "I fed my soul autumn color and light." The chapters are short, three or four pages; easy to read just one. But like a box of candy, one led to another, and to another, and then the next. I've saved a few for later, for the big chair by the fire. There is ice and snow out today, a perfect day for such a pleasure.

As a physician, I am aware that we exist in these bodies, as Judith portrays in her prayer that she might "…wear my furrowed, sun-dried body, with all of its life tracings . . . ." They define us in many ways, but we are more than our bodies. Her title, *Soul Medicine,* expresses this concept, and I suspect the purpose of these writings was in part to offer some healing. She is, after all, a physician.

Reading this caused me to remember things about myself, things I had forgotten, or had stored away as I was busy with the problems of life. In that remembrance I found some old joys, and found some old pains that had healed with time. I saw myself in these things she writes about. I put this book down, for now, with a greater peace than before. I had not expected that. I had not expected this book to be medicine for my own soul.

Jared L. Zeff, N.D., L.Ac.
January 4, 2016
Vancouver, Washington

INTRODUCTION

In my early twenties I spent four years outside the United States, living and traveling in Britain, India and Australia. I wanted to become a traditional medicine person, studying and practicing indigenous medicine. After living for a few months with traditional aboriginal people, I realized they had no reason to train someone in their medicine ways who was not committed to serving their people. I saw my dream of studying with a native healer as selfish if I had no plans of staying in the culture.

I turned to my own upbringing, searching for a form of medicine I could practice without selling my soul. I was grateful to discover naturopathic and Chinese medicines, both deeply rooted in the rhythms of the seasons and the elemental power of the Earth; however, my time living with indigenous people had taught me that even these medicines were incomplete.

I hungered for food and medicine for the soul as well as the mind and body. I wanted an elixir brewed with a respectful blend of local herbs, earnest prayer, and restorative community ceremony. I wanted medicines that were from and for the Earth, that supported the health and diversity of this body, my microcosm of the Earth, as well as the planetary body. I wanted medicine that nourished my whole being.

Over time I discovered the soul-restoring medicine of stories, gleaned from the heart and spoken like a poem or prayer. I began to cultivate my life, plowing the field of my experience, casting seeds of remembrance behind me and casting hope ahead, waiting for shoots to appear. I'd wander through these unfurling fields in moon-shadowed dreams, and tend them expectantly during the day. Gradually the fruits began to appear as short stories and reflections written and recorded for a weekly radio program, "The Mystic's Almanac."

The mystics are by definition an unstructured, formless society. Mystics discover divinity in the ordinary, in the simple and therefore easy-to-overlook moments that shape their daily rounds. Those who sought and discovered union with the divine often wore simple robes, not as a symbol of renunciation, but rather as a cover for the innate light they carried. The monks and nuns could not walk through a crowd without their internally generated light drawing the attention of those around them. The robes literally covered, and thereby protected, their illumination.

Now, in these transitional times, people are actively seeking those sparks of light. Many are awakening and discovering that light within them. Some have sought illumination for years. For others, awakening has arrived seemingly unbidden, with the crack of a soft-boiled egg at breakfast or the note of a bird at the window.

We live in a culture that no longer offers cloistered communities for those who are awakening to undergo these metamorphoses. We are being asked to transform in the midst of raising children, riding the subway, and making presentations at work. We alternately fumble and flourish, make leaps and lose our way.

Soul Medicine is food for the soul, to remind those awakening dreamers of their journey, and to offer nourishment along the Way. Writing offers the gift of standing in another's skin and looking through his or her eyes. From this privileged stance, I learn so much about the world and other human beings. Standing in another's shoes, I see myself more clearly.

Sun Bear, an Anishnabe elder who was a mentor and friend, helped me understand "medicine" is not a substance, like a pill or poultice, but rather *a way of living*. Healing might come from exotic plants or healing ceremonies. The most potent, sustainable medicines, though, arise from the stuff of daily life: interactions with our neighbors, plants that arrive unbidden in our gardens, the words spoken to a child in the last moments before sleep. These are the remedies that can change our lives and therefore our world.

These essays draw on earth-based wisdom. They are arranged according to the cycles of the year, starting with the winter solstice and continuing around the wheel of the year. Someone picking up the book in July, though, could easily set sail in the summer season. Many of the essays are universal and can be read at any time of the year. The seasonal sections are meant to provide gentle definition, not rigid separation, in the flow of the year.

More than anything I hope these essays will provide nourishment to other travelers, those who are making their own way and their own light in the world. May those seeking companionship discover a warm heart; may those searching for truth find light; may those praying for healing imbibe sweet medicine; and may those hungry for love discover deep nourishment. May you find this and much more in these pages.

WINTER

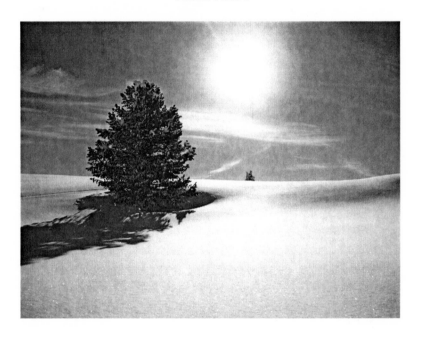

New Year's Resolutions

On the winter solstice, the darkest point in the wheel of the year, I plant seeds within myself. What do I want to nurture in the coming year?

In my mind's eye, I press a seed into the soil: more ease in my life. I pause in the wintery quiet. I press another seed into the slumbering earth: harmony, music; more time to play my violin.

This quiet vigil of planting seeds at the darkest point of the year feels more organic, and more sustainable, than making resolutions. A few years ago I unearthed one of my childhood journals. There, on January 1st, were my hopeful resolutions. I noted that the list had not changed much in the last 35 years. The "vices" I was hoping to correct were not life-threatening, yet my lack of success over nearly two generations startled me.

If I'm still struggling with the same issues that plagued me in childhood, what hope do I have of transforming the old and welcoming the new? Who do I know who has crossed that bridge, who has metamorphosed from caterpillar to butterfly?

For two years I worked at Portland Addictions Acupuncture Center in Oregon with people withdrawing from all kinds of drugs. I worked primarily with HIV+ and AIDS patients, some of whom were also recovering addicts.

One rainy winter afternoon I looked up from my charts to greet a new patient. A slender, muscular man with shoulder-length steely gray hair and a smooth, tanned face beamed down at me. His handsome face was familiar, but I couldn't place it right away.

"Hello," he said, extending a hand. "Will you be sticking me today?"

We both laughed. As he sat down beside me, my mind finally registered a hit.

"Is your name Tim?" I asked, picking up a chart.

"Yes," he said, surprised. "How did you know?"

"You probably don't remember me, but we were at a meeting together a couple of years ago."

He looked blank. I filled in the details about our volunteer work with a local Native American organization. I remembered him as a fast-talking business man, full of good ideas and the charisma to pull them off.

His face lit up. "Oh, yes, I do remember."

"And what brings you here today?"

Tim had contracted pneumonia two months earlier. He couldn't seem to shake the illness and finally ended up in the hospital. After a series of tests, he had been diagnosed with AIDS, with a T-cell count of 14. As a physician working with AIDS patients, I knew his immune system was barely functioning.

"I was living with my daughter, and also my fiancé, who's a lawyer," said Tim. "After the diagnosis, my fiancé left, and now my daughter is in foster care."

"I'm sorry," I told him.

He squeezed his eyes shut. "So am I."

Over the coming weeks, more of Tim's story gradually unfolded. He had been an athlete in high school, a native star rising in the small, eastern Oregon town where he'd grown up. He was also a drinker. His binges had worsened after high school, and he'd finally wound up in trouble with the law, eventually sentenced to Oregon State Penitentiary.

In the early '70s, Tim and another inmate instigated a riot. After the guards regained control, he and the other inmate were sent to a super-maximum security federal prison in Terre Haute, Indiana. Tim was facing life in prison, in one of the country's most oppressive penitentiaries.

While at Terre Haute, Tim kept up a steady correspondence. All of his pen pals were impressed by his intelligence and insight, and each wrote to the Oregon Parole Board asking that Tim be given the chance to rejoin society. Miraculously, after several years, the Oregon Parole Board consented to release Tim to live with a pair of elderly sisters in Washington State.

"When they released me from the prison," Tim recalled, "they drove me 10 minutes to the local Greyhound bus station. They paid for my ticket to Washington and gave me $25 traveling money, because I had nothing. I had 20 minutes to wait for the bus. There was a liquor store next to the bus station, and during those 20 minutes, I drank most of a fifth of vodka. I kept drinking all the way across the United States, until I arrived in Washington. The old ladies met me at the bus station. After about a month of staying with them, they told me they couldn't handle me anymore. I was totally out of control."

Tim next stepped onto a merry-go-round of drugs and women. He was in and out of Hooper, a residential detoxification center, four times.

"And then one night, I was in bed with my girlfriend, stoned on heroin or cocaine. I was lying there, and this feeling come over me.

"'Help me,' I said out loud. And a wave moved through me. I don't know if you would call it God or Spirit or what, but this feeling of grace passed through me. And I knew I would make it that time.

"I turned to my girlfriend and said, 'OK, I'm ready to go to Hooper.' She drove me to the detox center in the middle of the night. As we were walking up to the door, I stopped and said it again: 'Help me.' That feeling of grace came over me again."

He completed the residential program for the fifth time and never went back to drinking or taking drugs again.

I had worked at the addictions center just long enough to begin to see people cycling through for a second time. Through Tim's story, I began to see that more than willpower and intention determined their success or failure. What some might call "higher power," and what I would call grace, profoundly influenced the outcome of their efforts.

If intention and willpower were the primary currencies of creation, Tim would have been clean and sober years before his surrender to grace in front of Hooper. He had a rich bank account of intelligence and drive. The power of his mind, though, had to be coupled with some greater presence to ensure the metamorphosis he sought.

In the world of metaphysics, the law of attraction operates concurrently with the forces of chaos. When a patient berates herself for creating her illness, I ask her to consider a wind storm raging in a forest. Sometimes the strongest tree topples, while its decaying neighbor stands unscathed. That is the force of chaos at work, delivering its power blindly, like the scales of justice.

I can woo, but I cannot force creation. Enlightenment is by invitation only. I can prepare a room in my soul for a guest to enter, but I cannot force their occupancy. Their presence is by choice, an act of grace.

One episode of grace also does not guarantee another. Over the months I knew him, Tim's health continued to decline. The last time I saw him, his face and arms were deeply tanned, his smile peaceful.

"What have you been up to?" I asked, returning his smile.

"Fishing," he said quietly. "Spending hours every day on the banks of the Columbia River. I've been watching the light on the river. Always moving, always changing. That's what keeps me going – the light, the river."

Tim had come full circle, returning to the native roots of his ancestry, finding solace in the land, in the light, and within himself.

So I return to pressing seeds into the winter earth, in my mind planting the kernels of dreams as the wheel of the year turns anew. I will tend those seeds to the best of my ability, knowing that I must rely on the rains of grace to catalyze their growth.

The Face of Death

For over two years I traveled around the U.S. lecturing on menopause and women's health. Because I was constantly on the go, I carried a pager so that colleagues, friends, and family could reach me in case of emergency. My mom, unfamiliar with the technology, would call the number thinking she could reach me directly. "Mom," I told her as I returned one of her pages from an airport telephone, "I worry every time you page me. I think someone has died."

"Sorry, Honey," she crooned. "I just wanted to catch up with you and find out how you're doing."

A couple of months later, I was in a hotel room in Fort Worth, Texas, preparing to have dinner with one of my co-workers. The pager next to the bed began to vibrate and flashed a familiar number: my parents in Ohio.

I dialed, remembering my last conversation about the pager with Mom. My parents sounded tense and weary when they answered.

"Your sister Ruth was going in and out of consciousness this afternoon," said my mother, her voice as flat as a wind-swept prairie. My sister had recently had surgery to mend a badly broken leg, and I knew any surgery ran the risk of seeding a blood clot, especially in the leg. A blood clot could block the lungs, cause a stroke, or lodge in a major blood vessel.

"They took her to the hospital, and she died."

The words rolled through my brain and took all semblance of order with them. I groped for words, asked for details, and struggled to comprehend the enormity of losing the woman who was my closest biological and emotional link in the world.

I cancelled dinner plans and spent the evening crying and trying to choke down some room-service food. My sister was dead. My sister. Dead. The words kept rolling around in my mind, threatening to batter and destroy all of my carefully collected ideas about death and dying. I had counseled others about the power of death and the permanence of the soul. Death was the other side of life that created a sacred whole.

"At least I have some spiritual understanding of death," I

consoled myself, "which I'm sure will make the grieving process easier for me than the rest of my family."

That arrogant assumption haunted me over the coming years. As the numbness passed, anger replaced it. Why my sister? And where the hell was she? I expected to sense her in my daily life, converse with her in dreams, and generally continue to interact with her on "other levels." True to form, though, my sister exited quickly and cleanly. She was never one to linger or tarry. No doubt her Aries energy had catapulted her onward . . . to what?

Even my assumptions about past and future lives evaporated in the volcanic eruption of her sudden death. I was no longer certain what happened when someone died. Many times I thought of Ron Evans, a Chippewa-Cree teacher who shared a story about a native woman, raised in boarding school by Catholic nuns, who returned to Ron's reservation to discover her roots. She visited one of the elders, hoping to glean answers to spiritual questions from her own tradition that were as definitive as the catechism of her youth.

After a barrage of questions, she delivered her most urgent query last: "What happens when we die?"

The elder looked taken aback. "How would I know?" he asked. "I haven't died yet!"

I haven't died either, and up to that moment I had never looked death so directly in the face. What surprised me most was that death was expressionless. No joy. No tears. No judgment or celebration. Death was not masked, but rather faceless, smooth and unblemished.

Many years have passed since my sister Ruth's death. I have felt her presence only once, in a dream about Christmas Eve at the church we attended in our youth. Slowly I have come to new understandings of our voyage through and out of this life. I no longer believe that we have "life contracts" with specific entry and exit dates. I believe we have several points in our lives when we have the opportunity to leave, stay, and/or transform. I see now that my sister, with few worldly encumbrances, was ripe for a quick and easy exit.

I am reluctant to wrap explanations or conjecture around the experience of death. I want to leave space for the Mystery to inform me, in its ruthlessly magnificent way, about the mechanics of death.

The Face of God

My understanding of Spirit transformed following my sister's sudden passing just shy of her forty-first birthday. I have since learned that a beloved's death is often a major re-evaluation time in someone's life. Some meet grief stoically and use the experience to reinforce their theology. For others the passage through grief offers an opportunity to re-evaluate the landscape of belief, spirituality and faith.

I reflected on the maturation of my relationship with what I knew simply as "God" in my childhood. Even though I grew up in a Protestant church that eschewed images of divinity, I had developed a profile of God that was a cross between the white-skinned, lean-limbed old man of the Sistine Chapel and a department-store Santa Claus. The old white man transformed into an androgynous being during the feminist awakening of my junior-high-school years. As a teenager I spent several summers backpacking in wilderness areas, and during those trips I came to know the power of the creator through the beauty of nature. The singular face of God shattered, and each element of creation became a fractal of that magnificent life force. The creator metamorphosed again when I was a college student, becoming a purely feminine Goddess. I needed this womanly relationship with spirit to heal the centuries of patriarchy that have shaped contemporary Western religions. Years of contemplation and life in several spiritual communities once again softened the rigid gender designation, and my understanding of spirit resumed the diffuse, omnipresent divinity of my backpacking days. My work as a physician and acupuncturist further developed my experience of divine essence as I honed the ability to strengthen and move this godly life force or *qi*.

Throughout my spiritual journeying, my idea of *divinity* has remained rooted in the Earth and all of creation rather than a disembodied sky god lording over some celestial resort called heaven. I am most at home with ancient Tibetan traditions, my Shawnee family, and the spiritual roots of my Celtic ancestors who practiced the old ways of working with the underworld, the Goddess, and angelic beings. Divinity rests in the wilderness, the chapel, the garden, the bedroom, and my bones. When I am awake, Creator is alive in every aspect of my life.

My sister's death also uprooted my belief in a personal God. In retrospect I'm not sure how this concept of a cozy fairy godmother/father developed. Ruth's passing, in combination with another tragedy later that year, swept the remnants of a childhood God from my life. I suddenly understood that God does not stay up late at night worrying about the balance in my checking account. That is my job. Goddess is not plotting a career for me, repairing the roof, or inoculating my children against illness and tragedy. Creator had his/her own work and life to pursue: creating other worlds, playing golf, relaxing in a hot bath, whatever he/she wants to do.

When I recounted this realization to my Shawnee mentor, he nodded sagely. "Creator gave you life," he said, "and he/she, whatever you want to call it, gave you the ability to think and take care of yourself. That's your responsibility."

He paused for a moment, choosing his words carefully. "When I pray - and I do still pray - I ask for help in figuring something out. 'Creator, help me think through how to support my family. Help me figure out how to find a job.' You don't ask Creator to find the job for you, or give you the money. Life doesn't work that way. That would be insulting the intelligence Creator gifted you with. You pray as a capable person who needs help, not as a helpless being."

The Shawnee medicine man's words still guide me in my prayers. I continue to explore the essence of divinity. The shattering of old concepts has left a lot of uncharted territory, and I'm not terribly eager to replace one badly drawn map with another. Often I am uncomfortable in the new landscape; I like the security of a map. Even more, though, I am determined to see Divinity clearly. For now, Creator's face is as smooth and unblemished as Death's.

Bare Bones Landscape

Walking by the river today, as the sun rolled behind the rim of the Uncompaghre Plateau, I was dazzled by the contrast of snow against brown earth. In the late afternoon chill, I recognized the bare-boned soul of winter: hard ground, stark trees, and brittle grass. This landscape, dusty green in the summer, is now laid bare. I see animal traces I had never noticed in the weedy-green tangle of summer. The snow reveals those trails, as clear as tracings on the highway map.

Dog tracks follow the cement path in an even rhythm. Bird prints meander and then disappear, the moment of flight leaving no trace in the powdery stillness.

I see also a scattering of down, and the discarded tail feathers of a sparrow. From the surrounding marks in the snow, I know a hungry hawk found satisfaction in that place.

Just as the seasons turn, the wheel of the year revolving unceasingly from cold to thaw to blaze to decline, so, too, do we cycle as humans. In the spring of human life, we enter childhood with facile minds and quickly germinating bodies. Summer, or adolescence, is also marked by quick growth and the heat of emotional maturation. In our adult years, we harvest the autumnal fruits of our labor and begin to look inward for sustenance. Our elder years, marked with snowy white, are the season of giving away all that we have accumulated, physically, mentally, emotionally, and spiritually. We may give-away with agonized regret or joyous release. Willingly or woefully, in the winter of our lives we cast aside the old shell and prepare for new beginnings.

Now, in the cold bones of winter, I can see the traces, scars, and markings on the land. Everything is laid bare, with no vegetation to hide the marks.

I can see those same traces clearly outlined in the faces and bodies of beloved elders. Their bodies, their *earth*, carry the markings of their lives. Laughter has dug deep furrows around their eyes. Worry, deep listening, and concentration have plowed creases between their eyebrows. All of those emotions are recorded in the soft furrows of their earth.

On my own body, my fingers trace the faint thickening above my pubic bone where the surgeon's knife opened my boys' passage into the world. That line also marks the severing of my dream of a perfect birth, and our surrender to Creator's chosen path into this world.

I also have a scar cresting on my forehead, just at the hairline. At four years old, I fell backwards off a raised metal pool in a friend's back yard; my head landed on a pile of bricks. I walked home wailing, leaving a trail of bloody footprints on the driveway and the kitchen floor.

Those moments also left a trail in my body. I can feel the heat of that scar now, linking me to my sticky feet, my sour stomach, and my mother's shoulder encircling mine in the emergency room.

My body, like the winter snow, shows ever more clearly the trails I've taken. I have marks, scars, furrows, and depressions that mark my physical journey. Experience presses the soft clay of my flesh and shapes the bones and ligaments by force of habit, the vagaries of accidents, and dare I say "chance"?

Gradually, and I pray gracefully, this vehicle is passing away, returning to a bare bones landscape. I haven't entered my elder years yet; I'm tentatively approaching. As Caitlin Matthews says of her own menopausal journey, "I don't feel I have become a crone. That will happen when my bits start to drop off."

Winter reminds me of that final release in the utter simplicity of a snowy landscape. In this landscape, soft flesh meets hard-edged experience. I carry that marriage within me, every day. I can feel, and others can see, where the hard edges have snagged and shaped my form.

Someday I'll be plain, so gracefully simple, in my winter form. Stark white hair will flow over freckled skin, like fields of snow with sun-cleared patches. I admire the earth now, so sensuous in full surrender. I pray I may wear my furrowed, sun-dried body, with all of its life tracings, with equal grace.

My Refrigerator

My refrigerator is a repository of history, a living memorial to the ghosts of ancestors and housemates past.

Rummaging through the shelves I spy ancient sun-dried tomatoes packed in olive oil, left by a housemate who fled the West Coast for her native New Jersey almost four years ago. I discover a tiny bottle of "Jewelweed extract," a memento of my favorite housemate, a budding herbalist just entering medical school when she lived in the house. Next to the jewelweed sits a small plastic squeeze bottle with a film of massage oil lingering at the bottom, a relic that predates my move to this house. I wrapped the empty plastic bottle in my previous apartment seven years ago and moved it, unchanged, into my present refrigerator.

The top shelf houses a mostly empty jar of mayonnaise, a bottle of homemade salad dressing, several half-filled Mason jars, and a shiny holiday gift bag filled with seeds. This seed bag is a treasured gift from friends who moved to Hawaii. They knew these seeds meant for the clay soils and incessant rains of the Pacific Northwest would not flourish in tropical paradise. These friends have since moved back. I wonder if they would covet those seeds, seeing them so boldly displayed on the top shelf.

The second shelf is crammed entirely with seed packets of every description. Some of the commercial seeds were cast-offs from a school guidance counselor. Another plastic bag contains seeds in small manila envelopes scrawled with elegant printing, the gift of a patient with an equally fervent passion for gardening. A co-worker gifted me with a precious stash of heirloom seeds stored in unused "business reply mail" envelopes, with notes like "Bean — Amish Knuttle. Long, long vines — grow them up corn stalks." I have seeds from my mother, neatly labeled with name and year of collection. On the blue cornflower packet she added the message, "My Grandma Hibbert always had these in her garden and would pick a bouquet of cosmos, zinnias and cornflowers before we left." Several plastic bags hold seeds I have collected from my own garden. The rest are a motley assortment of organic seeds bought in moments of weakness at the health-food store or garden nursery. I have enough seed for several years of gardening.

Reluctantly I recognize a genetic tendency developing in myself that blossomed in full glory in my now departed great-aunt Loey. She was an immaculate housekeeper, a gene I did not inherit, and had a refrigerator full beyond reason for a single woman. The shelves were brimming with neatly arranged foodstuffs: a mustard jar harboring half a teaspoon of dried yellow crust, square jam jars covered with a thin film of purple stickiness, and catsup bottles with a dry, black ooze erupting around the cap. She scrawled messages on scraps of white paper and attached them to the condiment jars with rubber bands. They were reminders for recipes, or pleas for visiting guests to use the contents in an appointed meal.

I ponder the "save-it" allele, this genetic impulse that has been developing quietly over centuries in my family. I believe this gene resides close to the nesting instinct and the biological clock in my intricate helix of genetic material. This "squirrel" gene has evolved according to the demands of the times, its evolution spurred by centuries of war and famine and ill-fated economic times. The Great Depression of the 1930s added another layer of polish to this already dominant genetic tendency.

I live with the shadows of my ancestors so close to me. They haunt my love for seeds, my passion for gardening, and the slowly declining contents of my refrigerator. For you, Aunt Loey, tonight I'll eat a salad garnished with sun-dried tomato dressing. And I'll savor it with a bouquet of blue cornflowers on the table.

The Book Slut

Books are my lovers. My bed is littered with them, these paper tomes, and they leave no space between the covers for a human mate to settle.

Books have befriended me since I was a child. Much of my childhood was lost to illness. Often, when I was sick, I was too feverish to concentrate on reading. When I was able, though, I devoured books. The reading seemed more restorative than the many rounds of antibiotics and other drugs I swallowed. I remember reading *Ramona the Pest* during a two-day siege of the stomach flu. I finished the book at 8:30 p.m. on the second day. I knew I would have to return to school the next morning, and I couldn't bear to leave the book unfinished, like a conversation dangling in mid-sentence.

Sometimes I lost myself completely in books, even when I wasn't ill. Once, as a ten-year-old, I parked myself under a shady tree at the local pool and fell into a volume of *The Three Investigators* series. Two hours later one of the neighbor girls stood beside me, shouting.

"*Judith!*" she screamed. Her face was red, her voice hoarse. "I've been yelling at you for two minutes!"

Dazed, I looked up into the summer sunshine. I hadn't even been aware of the book, much less the people milling around the pool. The story had completely taken me, like the proverbial magic carpet, into some other realm.

From college on, I lived primarily in the world of non-fiction. I studied some literature in college, but the majority of my reading was devoted to music, science, religion, and philosophy. After graduation I decided to shift my focus from book education to life education. I wanted life itself to woo me with its teachings. Of course, I still had some clandestine affairs with literature, such as *Woman on the Edge of Time* and *The Color Purple*. The community where I lived at the time was decidedly anti-intellectual, so I had no compatriots in whom I could confide my indiscretions. The covert nature of the affair was bittersweet — tantalizing but lonely.

After six years of life education, I returned to medical school. I discovered once again the joy of reading. I had too many weighty texts to indulge in the "frivolous" world of fiction.

During one holiday break, though, I picked up a Barbara Kingsolver novel from the local library. I traveled to Ohio to visit my family. One afternoon I developed a low-grade fever. I crawled into my childhood bed at 2 p.m. and picked up the only book I had with me, *Animal Dreams*. I fell into that book, and I fell hard. In love. Deeply in love. I had forgotten how deeply nourishing fiction could be. Non-fiction feeds my mind; fiction feeds my soul. The story was good, the writing great. I had another frisson of recognition: I had discovered a new writer, and this meeting promised to be a long-term love affair. At 2 a.m., 12 hours after opening the book, I finished the last page and turned off the light. My fever was gone.

I eagerly await new Kingsolver novels, just as lovers might await a delicious rendezvous. When the new novel arrives, I know I will have to ration myself so that I don't stay up too late and stumble bleary-eyed into the clinic the next day, physically torpid but emotionally sated from the tryst.

I haven't read the last two Harry Potter books because I know I would lose at least two days of work. I'd have to call patients and make lame excuses, ferry my children off to babysitters, and then sequester myself somewhere until the book had had its way with me. The machinery in some novels is just too strong to resist. I know certain books have the power to ensnare me so completely that I just don't go near them, and Harry Potter rates among those forbidden fruits.

The greatest privilege of reading, whether fiction or non-fiction, is to go walkabout in someone else's mind. I know of nothing more intimate than the deep sharing of mental territory, the exploration of someone else's life terrain. Through writing, we meet in ways that even the most intimate body contact cannot duplicate.

And amazingly, like that epiphany in my childhood bedroom, we make these discoveries in private, long after the author has scrawled a map of the territory, and the smoking trail of the pen has gone cold. Sometimes we peer hundreds, if not thousands of years into time and discover the mind-stuff is just as fresh and vital as the seeds excavated in the pyramids. These mental walkabouts allow me to move in territories that are both contemporary and ancient, with equal ease. I have the privilege of looking through someone else's eyes, standing in her shoes, stretching inside his skin. Their whole world opens deeply, intimately to me. If the encounter is good, I count them as friends. If the terrain is transformative, I take them as lovers.

With all of the paper lovers inhabiting my bed, no wonder I have spawned paper babies (i.e. books) myself. I've caught the fever of wanting to share my mental terrain with others, perhaps hoping to return the favor of a pleasure I have so deeply enjoyed.

I notice my boys have adopted a similar habit. When they have fallen deeply in love with a book, they beg to tuck it under their pillow at night. I know of no higher compliment to pay a book than to take it to bed. I smile when I see a new book stashed like clandestine treasure under a pillow, with one of the boys peacefully sleeping on top. Sweet dreams, little one. I know you're becoming a book slut, too.

Blood Mysteries

My blood runs blue today, as scarlet poppies bloom between my legs. After a couple of weeks of crescendo, the tension building in my breasts and womb like a drawn bow, that tautness is loosed, the bow string slack. My sharply focused mind relaxes in tandem with my unfurling womb. Body and soul surrender to this lunar rip-tide.

In native cultures, I would be strolling to the moon hut now. I would not be banished from the village, but rather welcomed into the sanctuary of women. In this quiet, dreamy space, away from the incessant demands of children, a mate, a practice, I could allow that slack, un-pointed mind to go walkabout, to dream, to create, and to prophesy.

The veils between the worlds are thinnest when the first spot of blood darkens the toilet paper. I sigh with relief, celebrating the freedom of my womb. PMS and early pregnancy are so difficult to differentiate. Since my late teens I have prayed for these ruby spots on my underpants, banners to announce my unfurling womb. This month I will not hold my blood. I will not plant a seed within the bloody velvet of my uterus. No, I will allow it to flow freely, in achy spurts, from my soft-bellied womb.

Only on a few rare occasions have I been able to deeply relax into my moon-time dreaminess. Once my blood began to flow as I descended into the Haleakala Crater. Fasting, I walked eleven miles across that slumbering volcano, then planted myself in the damp rainforest on its far rim.

For three more days I wandered in the belly of the crater. Already altered by hormonal tides, I entered much more deeply into pools of meditation. I experienced my womb as the seat of my creativity. If I could imagine and shape my life from this creative core, I knew the power of my life creations would be beyond measure.

So today, with summer sun blazing, I retreat inward, into the lunar eclipse that is my belly. In this soft, achy twilight, I surrender to moon-minted wisdom.

As a woman, the moon influences my life more than the sun. For men, the solar cycle offers a steady monotony – sunrise, peak, sunset, darkness. The days vary in length, but the daily alteration is almost imperceptible. In this male-identified world, I am expected to adhere to this solar pattern, behaving and appearing the same way from day-to-day.

As a woman, I feel the moon wooing the watery tides I carry within me – blood, saliva, lymph. I feel the moon growing in my belly. If I lived without other nocturnal light, that tide would crest at full moon, when my almond-shaped ovaries would release an egg that would sail into the fluttering arms of the Fallopian tube. For two weeks that egg would journey down that tunnel, passing through darkness as the moon wanes, feasting on herself until she is a thin rib, and then nothing more. If fertile, that egg would nestle into the moist velvet of the womb, and begin its slumbering journey to creation.

Other lunar months, the egg enters this dark, wet emptiness as a barren seed. The fertile dress begins to unravel, taking the seed with it as it passes in shreds into the outer world.

My womb most likely will never "hold blood" to shape another human life. Instead, those seemingly barren seeds pass into the world as the progeny of dreamtime – ideas, soft-formed and growing; projects, still fresh with wet velvet on their wings. When I surrender fully to the bloody darkness in the womb, prophecy emerges – whispers of the future and glimpses of the past.

I'm not sure how many more turns of the lunar cycle I will continue to dance. The rhythm is increasingly erratic. The moon seems to be softening her firm hold on my inner tides. Eventually I will move to a rhythm more majestic than sun or moon. When the lunar tides, so compelling in their waltzing beat, quiet in my womb, I will move to stellar rhythms, as the night-sky continues to orbit within me – slow drum beats, reverberating over millennia.

Increasingly my cadence is internal, as star-cycles trump the moon's. No matter the rhythm-maker, though, the womb will continue to be the reverberating throne of my creativity.

Death Poem

Joe arrived at the clinic in a T-shirt and faded jeans. He was considering a transition from life in the Arizona desert to the mountains of Colorado. He had driven Colorado's narrow mountain highways 30 years before as a truck driver. Later in life Joe had returned to school to study acupuncture, mastered his craft, and then began to teach. Somewhere along the journey he had unearthed the mystical roots of his Jewish heritage and mixed that soulful brew with the river of Taoist thought. Ill health had truncated his teaching career. He was scheduled for a surgery to remove one kidney, and his wife planned her departure, as well.

Despite all of the changes and transformations that lay before him, Joe approached this crossroads with witty composure. After returning home, he sent an e-mail to friends announcing his newly chosen home: "Many places qualify as 'God's Country,'" he wrote, "but Colorado is where Yahweh vacations."

The recovery from surgery was much longer and rougher than Joe expected. He sent erratic e-mails, and I made occasional phone calls during his recovery. After several months, Joe moved to Colorado. The trip taxed his already fragile body, and he immediately landed in the hospital.

Despite spending almost half his days in dialysis, Joe launched a website, choosing a new moniker for himself: the simple country acupuncturist. This humble offering, though, belied a profound depth of knowledge. Joe offered to teach me the pain-relief technique he had perfected, but I was beginning my own transition. When the planned date arrived, I already was on a riptide headed east, to a new home in Oklahoma.

Ten days ago an e-mail arrived from Joe, marked "The Simple Country Acupuncturist: Last Post." Joe, true to his Taoist roots, was offering his final wisdom. He was stepping into a venerable stream that has flowed through many centuries. In Japan *jisei*, or death poem, is a gift to one's friends, students and loved ones. Often these final thoughts are particularly lucid. Some shine with wisdom, others with humor.

I share with you Joe's final words, that you, too, might bask in the wisdom gleaned from his life journey, walking with one foot in the Kabbalah and the other in the Tao:

"This will be my last post. A slow separation of my Yin & Yang has begun. My body is heavy and its movements unsure. Inside my spirit is light and gathering in my upper Jiao. When I go outdoors I feel the touch of the sky in my chest and the Yang currents in my arms. I will enter hospice in a few days. My scholarly acuity is now intermittent and this piece will not have the fluidity I strive for. But elegance is not the goal. It only makes a good thought more communicable and disseminates it further.

"There are so many things I could talk about with you but time is of the essence and so I have tried to choose the most important. I haven't done a methodical examination of all the candidates but after a bunch of thought, right now, today, I believe the most important of all human characteristics to be empathy.

"Empathy is the first spark of the tenderness holding an infant evokes. It is the urge to put a comforting hand on a friend's shoulder. It enables us to understand some of another person's motivations. And sadness and frustrations. It allows us to recognize a fellow in an enemy. It allows us to forgive a wrongdoer, to give a second chance. Empathy is why we volunteer for the sake of others. Why we make contributions to good causes. Empathy is the prototype of our gentle emotions.

"Empathy motivated the group of people who didn't know me at all to get up extra early or take time from their work day to get me to and from dialysis for two months. And it was the force that motivated my extraordinary friend YM Chen to bring me greetings and succor from friends and colleagues.

"Empathy is the core impetus of the Golden Rule. And the Golden Rule is the dialectical opposite of cynicism. It is the preservative and constructive Yang force to the destructive and entropic Yin force. The kindness we desire, given to others, is the balancing entity to man's inhumanity to man."

The Sephardi Taoist
February 4, 2013

[The message that Joe had passed arrived 15 minutes after completing this essay.]

Animal Love

Lions, when they mate, spend 24 hours a day sleeping and making love. They do not hunt but rather feed on the ecstasy of flesh meeting flesh, fur tangling in moist fur. They awake only to enjoy the pleasure of each other's tawny bodies. The male roars when he comes, spilling his seed into the female, then licking her clean.

Eagles mate in midair, soaring thousands of feet above the Earth before locking talons and free-falling, screaming with pleasure, parting only a few feet from the ground. They narrowly avoid death in the creation of new life. The French call orgasm "the little death." Eagle knows the dual-hinged door between life and death swings both ways.

Salmon live by a passion for place, an urge that magnetizes them from a distance of hundreds, sometimes thousands of miles, a memory that endures from hatchling days, perhaps even from the moment the ovum first cleaves into a two-celled being. Salmon exhaust themselves on the journey, spending the last of their strength laying eggs and then baptizing them with sperm. The tail fin waves over the eggs like the arms of a priest swinging his censer over the altar, fertilizing the soulful congregation with clouds of smoldering myrrh. Salmon, too, know death in the creation of life, more intimately than Eagle, who merely flirts at the doorway but does not pass through the portal.

I love you like an animal.

I love you with my body as well as my heart and soul. Like animal: simple, powerful, direct. I love your juices, your fur, your flesh. I love the curve of your muscles, the wetness of your tongue, the downy curls of your hair. I love your scent and the warmth that radiates from your body in the early morning hours as we lie moonstruck under summer sheets.

Like Lion, I could feed for days on nothing but the ecstasy of your flesh and fur, the moist places that hold the secret of our love.

Like Eagle, you take me to the edge of death, free-falling into places I have not known, or that have slumbered in a dreamy past.

In that "little death" I am dying to a way of life that no longer suits me: the death of loneliness, of isolation, of separation from sources of strength. I am finding a new life, homing to some place I do not consciously remember.

Did I know when I was conceived, even before the first splitting of the ovum, the shape of your face, the texture of your hair, the curve in the river that is your arms? Did I memorize the color of your eyes and the sound of your voice before I ever moved through the dual-hinged door of life and death?

I'm coming home to the source of my life, the end of a long journey, to cast my seed and die to a new way of life.

Meet me in the waters.

This is your home, too.

On Loan

Today I stopped at the library to choose books and a new video for my twin toddler boys. I was once a member of a children's book-of-the-month-club but my wallet has now grown too thin to justify anything more than necessities: baby-sitters, organic bananas, and malpractice insurance.

I think of my mom driving us kids to the library. I learned how to write my name when I was four years old so that I could have my own library card. Mom knew how to stretch $1,000 over a year to support a family of five. The library was part of that miracle.

Tonight, I bring home another stack of books. I feel the same excitement I did when I unwrapped packages from the children's book club. The only difference is that the books are free (as long as I return them on time), a loan against all of our taxpayers' generosity. I marvel at the whole concept of libraries. Some creative genius envisioned this resource: free and open to the public, treasures of knowledge for all who would avail themselves.

On loan, yet the boys' excitement lasts about the same length of time whether the book is bought or borrowed. They greet my arrival with excited squeals. I drop the books in the front hallway and then begin to prepare dinner. I catch sight of one of them sitting in the corner carefully, even lovingly, turning the pages.

On loan. So I tell the boys to be more careful with these books. "These are not *our* books," I explain. "We have to treat them extra nicely because they're borrowed."

On loan. I think of Kalil Gibran and his great teaching about children in *The Prophet:*

Your children are not your children.
They are the sons and daughters of Life's longing for itself.
They come through you but not from you,
And though they are with you yet they belong not to you.

On loan, my children are. Do I remember to treat them more carefully, more kindly, than something that "belongs" to me? How easily I fall into thinking I own my children. As a single mom, aren't I the breadwinner, primary comforter, boundary-maker, head priestess, poopy-diaper washer, "owie" kisser, and punching bag? Don't I have controlling interest in this common stock known as "my sons"?

No. Like the generous library system that trusts me to return common property, Creator has loaned me two souls to nurture. In my best moments, I treat the boys with extra deference. They belong to the public of souls, the commonwealth of spirit. I need to return them in good condition. I pray that any "wear" will be from pats and snuggles and howling tickle fights. I pray that I will return these boys well-read (from careful listening), well-worn (from fond handling) and well-loved.

If I Were a Beautiful Woman

For weeks now I have agonized over a former lover's rejection of my body.

"I wish I could take you out and buy you some clothes," he had said, eyeing my half-clad body carelessly wrapped in a bath towel. "You could look so beautiful."

I'd stared at him. Droplets of bath water fell from my long, golden hair onto the wooden floor, beads that could have been tears had my heart been beating. The words still shock me. *Could* be beautiful? And what was wrong with me the way I was?

"I mean, you could wear short skirts, not really short, just up to here," he'd said, sketching a line with his hand about 10 inches above my knee.

Why did his words cut so deeply, I wondered? Hadn't I learned to love my body, to stop the agonized wishing that I could weigh 125 pounds like every 5 foot 11-inch model parading through the pages of *Vogue* magazine?

So, when had I begun the quest for beauty, the search for the holy plastic grail? I joined the "World of Beauty" club at age 12, thinking I would discover beauty in the box of products that was to arrive each month, but I cancelled my membership after two months. The Nail Strengthener, fluorescent blue eye shadow, and under-eye cover-up brought me no closer to the Grail.

I started wearing a bra when I was in the fourth grade, the first girl in my class to don her training gear. The other kids taunted my fledgling signs of puberty. At 11 and 12 they jeered again when I chose not to wear a bra, a show of defiance as I joined my older sisters who were proclaiming their full breasted freedom to swing and bounce uninhibited.

I shaved my legs a couple of times during the fourth grade, again before the other girls in my class did. That summer, my next door neighbor's brother made a big point of complaining when the newly re-sprouted hairs brushed against his bushy legs. Later, when all the other girls were scraping the hair off their legs and underarms, I discarded my razor – out of sync again.

The summer of my 13th year, one of my favorite camp counselors cornered me on the archery range. "When are you going to cut down those fur trees?" he asked, pointing at my legs.

I looked at the soft, golden down on my legs and flinched. Without a word, I went back to the cabin and borrowed my sister's razor. I escaped to the shower room, soaped my legs, and began to drag the blade over my skin. I accidentally gashed my lower shin, leaving a scar that remains to this day, a reminder of the self-mutilating ritual that I have never again repeated.

Always I have been too early or too late, too bold or too tame, never meeting someone else's elusive definition of beauty. I remember a summer romance with a mathematics professor at Indiana University, and his unfailing shock that I wasn't involved with some hot-testicled college male. "You're so beautiful," he told me. "You must be putting out a message that you don't want to be involved with anyone."

And perhaps I was. I was recovering from a heart rent by my ex-fiancé, who had left me for a bassoonist, a full-bodied woman with dark hair shaped by the inherited refrains of Mediterranean sunlight in her blood. She, too, was everything I was not.

I am coming to the inescapable conclusion that beauty must be internally defined if it is to mean anything, yet that definition has been culturally influenced. Almost everyone gasps at the same moment in response to a particular image projected on the screen. We all have similar lenses, ground by the constant cultural grist of media exposure.

Those lenses are modified by religious and academic training, by the passing fancies of magazine editors and fashion designers, by the co-option (and thereby trivialization) of grassroots counter-movements. As Annie Dillard notes, the one-celled organism, lacking the complex neural functions that create cultural lenses, probably sees the world most purely.

In the end, though, beauty is more than pure seeing. Beauty comes from seeing with loving eyes, from placing oneself in relationship with the object of one's gaze.

All of my lovers have been beautiful to me. Some were fat,

some had straggly hair, some had furry backs, some were drop-dead handsome, but all were beautiful.

Love is blind, the cynic declares. Love to me, though, refocuses the eye. When I see with loving eyes, I witness beauty that otherwise lies dormant, perhaps hidden to the casual observer.

In love, I am not blind. I see the divine in the disheveled, the grace amidst the grit, the elegance in the aged. Love opens my eyes to celebrate beauty in the overlooked, the angular, and the unexpected. Love transforms my eyes.

The House of Marriage

I inhabited the house of marriage for five years. When my husband became abusive and we separated, my mother reminded me of a story Garrison Keillor told about a woman who left Lake Wobegone on the train bound for Chicago. When the train pulled into the station, the woman put her hand on her son's knee. "Imagine that!" she exclaimed. "We're in Chicago!"

I stared blankly at my mother.

"You know, you get on the train to Chicago, what do you expect when it arrives?" she asked dryly.

That was her polite way of saying, "I told you so."

For the last four-and-a-half years, since embarking on the journey of being a single parent, I've been reflecting on the structure of marriage. How did I choose and then construct a marriage? How did I manage to draw up blueprints for a "house" to inhabit that was so antithetical to my previous life, and my innate way of being?

Now, if I built a house that didn't suit me, no one would think any less of me for putting it on the market and moving elsewhere. In this culture, though, the expectation is that we humans move two by two, like animals herding toward some imaginary ark, the presumed salvation from a flood of . . . what? Emotion? Financial destitution? Loneliness? Insecurity?

The same mother who delivered the artful "I told you so" story also overlooked introducing me at her fortieth wedding anniversary. I'm not certain whether the omission was conscious or not, but along with a widowed neighbor, I was the only single adult woman in the room. Seated in the back corner with my unwed teen-aged nephews, I'm certain I was a disappointment to my mother. Sadly, she was no happier with my chosen groom.

How *did* I end up choosing my husband? I remember grappling with a similar question when I was 25 years old, recovering from surgery in a hospital in India. The staff chose a bed for me next to a village woman who knew a few words of English. Together with my 20 words of Tamil, we were able to carry on rudimentary conversations.

"You may choose your husband, no?" Garidja asked me one day.

"Yes," I nodded.

"So who is he?" she asked. Most Indian parents arrange marriages for their children by the time they are three or four years old. The older women in the hospital ward looked at me with pity in their deep, brown eyes. At twenty-five, I was far beyond marriageable age. I was also without any family, an unthinkable situation in India, where family members bathe, cook for, feed, and toilet an ailing relative. The hospital nurses' primary duty is dispensing medication, not caring for patients.

After 20 minutes of heated conversation, I finally realized Garidja assumed I knew who my husband would be, and I was simply traveling around the planet until I was ready to tie the knot. She was angry that I would not tell her the name of my betrothed.

"Garidja, I don't know who my husband will be."

Her anger faded to confusion. "How do you choose?"

Her question startled me. How did I decide?

"Um, we date."

"Date? What is 'date'?"

"Well, you spend time together, go to movies, take walks, get to know each other."

Garidja stared hard at me. I realized this was like explaining sex to a Martian. We had more than language as a barrier between us. "But how do you decide?"

Her question has haunted me for nearly 20 years. How did I, or anyone in this culture, make such a momentous decision? I realized most of my training came from fairy tales. Prince and princess meet, look into each other's eyes, fall madly in love, marry, and "live happily ever after." The decision is based purely on emotional and physical chemistry. The tales give no direction on how to build a solid, long-lasting structure for that marriage to inhabit. We never see the couples arguing over TV channels, money, or methods for disciplining children. They remain forever in newly wedded bliss.

Most of Asia relies on a polar-opposite method. Bride and groom often have never met before they stand together at the altar. What love they share will be cultivated, carefully grown over years, rather than the result of spontaneous combustion.

When I first arrived in India, I considered the local marriage customs barbaric. How could any thinking person agree to marry someone he or she had never even seen before? Gradually, though, I began to discern wisdom in the marriage arrangement. The villages relied on a carefully constructed social order to survive. Most individual families thrived with clearly defined roles and expectations. Certainly not every family was harmonious; alcoholism and abuse were present in about the same percentages as in the West (albeit more visible and audible in the windowless village houses.) I began to see that my Western ideas could potentially topple an artfully balanced order that had evolved over millennia.

Even more disturbing was the realization that the cultivated, slow-growing love that an arranged marriage engendered might actually be more durable than the hormonally driven, hot-house approach we relied on in the West. In public, Indian couples rarely touched. I had witnessed, though, an Indian husband caressing his wife's bare shoulder as she stooped over the cooking fire, in the privacy of their own home. Their affection was palpable. And sustainable.

Who was I to criticize the arranged marriage when, for some, the method worked as well or better than my own?

With the experience I have accrued, what sort of a marriage would I build now? I've dabbled once with dating; I've mentally courted a partnership. Sometimes I've moaned to friends about my singular life with my twin boys. During one of my angst-ridden reflections about relationships, one of my mentors challenged me.

"Judith, you haven't even asked if it's appropriate for you to be in a relationship."

I was stunned. For years I had fought the social conditioning that everyone (especially *women*) needed to be in a relationship. Not just any relationship, but a partnership. A marriage to be exact. I had not realized how deeply I had been socialized. I had unconsciously adopted the attitude that without a mate to march with me, two-by-two, I was going to miss my ride on the ark (and hence, salvation).

"You know, there are lots of wonderful people who have chosen *not* to have a partner," she continued. "Look at the Dalai Lama. He doesn't have a partner. Look at what he is doing in the world."

My mind reeled. I knew that she was right. I didn't *need* a husband. I know some men and women who absolutely function better with a mate. The truth, though, was that I was whole and complete, with or without a mate. I had not recognized that fulfillment in myself before. And in that moment I regretted all of the time I had spent fretting about relationships.

What if I could reclaim all of the evenings I had spent with girlfriends commiserating about our fate as single women? What if I could cash in every oracular device I had consulted about when, where, and who my next partner would be? What if all of the energy I had expended worrying about relationship could be redeemed?

Sometimes I imagine that I can shape-shift back in time and leave messages for my younger self. If I could make the journey, I would tell myself at twenty-one, heartbroken about a philandering fiancé, to save my energy for more important things. "You are strong and creative and numinous," I would tell that blossoming woman. "Don't let his actions blight your sapling limbs. Keep growing. You have so many seasons yet to greet."

And I would visit my thirty-year-old self and tell her that the green vines of her newly sprouting career would sustain her better than any hot-house lover. And I would tell my thirty-five-year-old self to heed all of the dreams that warned her about her husband-to-be.

And what messages would I seed for my future self? Build a house that suits you. Choose your companions with care. Leave plenty of space in the yard for your maturing limbs to spread and catch the sun. Enjoy your children. Keep your sense of humor. Stop waiting for Prince Charming to appear. Leave the door open for an appropriate mate to enter. And most importantly, stop waiting for a husband so you can "get on with your life." Your life is happening right now. There's too much life pulsing in you to feel alone. Let your home be the world. Let life inhabit you.

Sonja Bullaty

"I was fourteen-and-a-half exactly," said Sonja Bullaty, "because that's when Hitler came to Prague, and I was thrown out of school. That was the end of my formal schooling. My father was wise enough to give me a Rolleiflex camera. I absolutely loved it. So it was long before the horror came that I was introduced to photography. And it was the one thing that I was able to come back to."

In October 1941, on her 16th birthday, Sonja was taken to Auschwitz, one of the most notorious of the Nazi concentration camps.

"And then it was four years," said Sonja. "Strangely enough, I always thought that I was going to live, which is crazy. It's insane. There was just no reason for me to have survived, except a total fluke. Since 1941 I feel I've been given a gift.

"On the day I was released, it was ghastly, and it was wonderful. It was just like much of my life, total extremes. It was absolutely marvelous that you are alive, that you are facing a living future, and horrendous because there is no future, because there is no one to go back to. I walked out of the camp determined to prove to myself that life is beautiful, and despite everything to the contrary, that there are people worth loving.

"I had a friend who was Polish, whom I had met in the camp, and the two of us went to Prague, even though she was Polish. We slept on the floor of a school. I couldn't face going back to the family apartment.

"There is an old synagogue in Prague, where they have written out the names of all the people who had perished, just from Prague alone – over 79,000. In small letters, from ceiling to floor, are the names, in alphabetical order. I made myself read a lot of the names. And I think it was then that I finally accepted those people really weren't going to come back. But as long as I was in Prague (right after my release), I believed that the war wasn't over yet, and I would go chasing after who I thought was my mother, or friends, only to realize they were of course not them."

Sonja apprenticed herself to the Joseph Sudek, the preeminent

Czechoslovakian photographer of that time. Sudek had lost an arm during World War I, and he reclaimed his life through photography. He began by photographing trees.

After her release from the concentration camp, Sonja also was drawn to photograph trees. "They were the best friends I had," explained Sonja. "They would grow, they would fall and be half broken or struggling. I felt a really close kinship with the struggling ones. But the amazing thing is they would break out and bloom in the springtime. The whole idea that there was a next springtime, after whatever (horror), that whole metamorphosis to me was reassuring."

Sonja joined the orbit of musicians and photographers circling around Sudek, "the poet of Prague." Distant relatives eventually found Sonja's name among the list of survivors and invited her to live with them in New York City. Sonja left Prague for Paris, with the intention of continuing on to the United States. Her three-day jaunt in Paris stretched to three months.

Traveling through Germany, her train was derailed. Because of the delay, Sonja arrived in Paris 24 hours late, and no one was waiting for her at the station. One of the passengers who had shared her train compartment found Sonja an attic room to stay in. Sonja lived on baguettes and soup from the refugee kitchens. For three months, until her money ran out, she roamed the streets, photographing Paris.

Although the women where she lived were "very nice," they told her she could not come back to her room until after hours, close to midnight. "It took me years to figure out where I had been living," said Sonja, laughing. "It was a whorehouse."

Sonja left Paris for New York City, where she soon met her husband Angelo. "His life wasn't an easy one, either. He had been photographing trees. It was really the trees in some way that gave back to me, because Time-Life saw our photographs of trees throughout the seasons. We were involved in their first series of wilderness books. So the trees gave me the gift of employment," she said.

Later that night Sonja, Angelo, and I walked along the snowy streets and boarded one of the city buses. Less than a week before Christmas, the storefronts were festooned with lights and decorations.

"Oh, look!" exclaimed Sonja, jumping from her seat and stumbling across the moving bus for a better look at one of the displays. She turned and beamed at me with absolute joy. I broke into a grin.

She staggered across the moving bus and dropped into the seat next to me. "All the people on the bus think I'm a tourist," she said rolling her eyes, "because I get so excited. I've lived here almost 40 years, and I'm still in love with it."

Sonja was quiet for a few moments; then, she gently touched my arm. "It is a gift that we are able to see. I feel that we are more blessed than lots of people who don't, because we are given an extra dimension. It's like there are people who are musical, and people who aren't, and I think the ones who don't hear music are losing a great deal. It's the same with the visual, that you are given an additional life.

"It's not the equipment, it's *you* who takes the pictures. It is your communication with whatever the subject matter is, whether it's a person or a landscape or a flower or a cat. It's your rapport, your relationship to it – that is the only thing that matters. I'm very uncomfortable with manipulated pictures. I tend to resent them because I think our world is so incredibly beautiful, and it has not been explored enough as it is. I don't want to interfere with my vision. I prefer clean, one-to-one, whatever I'm with.

"That is, I think, one of the great gifts in life. To see something wonderful, and to know that it's wonderful. Just like when you have some relationship that is wonderful, and to know it's wonderful. Lots of people go through life taking things for granted. They live in a wonderful place, they have a happy family, or whatever, but they don't know it. Only when it's gone will they know it, and then it's too late. So, aren't I lucky," she asked, leaning forward and whispering, "I *know*."

SPRING

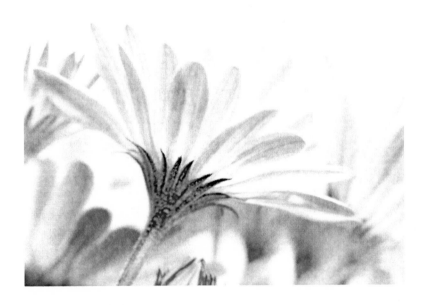

Jitterbug Spring

Spring is no retiring maiden. She's the seasoned dancer with creased leather boots, cherry-red, and scuffed. She's the one on the dance floor, stomping and spinning, her heels a molten blur. She's moist and fragrant with the scent of sweat. This is the movement of youth – eager, nimble, tireless. Spring is break-dance season, all tumble and hop and spin. No refined tango of summer or rhythmic waltz of autumn. No, this is youthful, spontaneous movement, all percussion and staccato saxophone. This is movement that takes over the body and makes a celebration of the limbs.

Summer skates. Autumn strolls, winter slides . . . and spring jitterbugs in my soul.

This is the season of air, the ground-shaking winds that thrum the house and set it vibrating. The trees bow and sway and break, any brittleness torn away in the apocalyptic power of the spring winds.

Ending the old, ushering in the new. This is Shawnee New Year, the fertile seed of newness planted in the icy heart of winter. This is the beginning of growth so stubborn, so inspired, that it sprouts amidst the detritus of the autumn and the snowy remnants of winter.

Wind defines spring, a relentless movement of air that carves rock and stirs the earth with newness. Spring wind is the hormonally driven surge of youth, ripping all that is extraneous from the winter-brown earth. Branches, limbs, shingles, buckled boards and rotting fence posts succumb to this transformative blast. Opening the land, laying bare all that is strong and fertile, the winds surge and cleanse.

I stand in the blast as long as I dare, then wrestle the door closed as the wind chimes brawl with the winds. Anything loose tosses restlessly, then surges into the whirling winds. Gone are the cardboard boxes, the rubber ball, the empty flower pots awaiting seedlings. Gone with the wind. Gone with the tidal wave of air that defines this season of growth.

How much energy the wind needs to wrest life from the jaws of winter, to catalyze the frozen Earth, to warm and woo it back to life. Spring is both growth and death, the meeting of these opposing forces. Spring and autumn are the pivotal linchpins of the year, the insistent note in a Beethoven symphony, at first dissonant, that becomes the defining note of a new movement.

Spring moves at a frenzied pace. I find hints of the green world stirring in the gravel – embryonic dandelion leaves among the rocks. The pussy willows press slivers of cotton from their brown-skinned buds – all accented with snow in the grey early-morning light.

The winds of warmer weather weave between the snowy days, teasing me with thoughts of sandals and sleeveless dresses. For now, though, the winds still cut into my skin, warning me that soft-skinned creatures still need protection. I know spring has fully arrived when wind moves around instead of through me.

This is the season when I discard the debris of living – ash from the wood-burning stove that has settled on every surface; old books and papers; orphaned socks and tattered clothes; children's shoes cracked and broken with wear.

The house inhales as the windows creak in their sashes and the doors swing open to allow the cleansing breezes to flutter the curtains and tease the dusty piles of papers. These winds are stirring the remnants of a life I am irrevocably leaving. These are the winds tousling last season's leaves, as surely as they dance among the supple spring-green shoots.

The winter calls me inward, to nurture seeds planted in the velvety darkness of a night sky. Now, in spring, wind invites me to dance, to jitterbug, to entice those wintery seeds into quick growth.

I breathe on these wintry seeds, and gently tap on the sodden cover of last autumn's leaves. This drumming stirs the slumbering earth, the swelling seeds.

I'm drumming, drumming, inviting the dance of newness in my life. Tapping, tapping, I'm stirring the dance of spring in the soil and in my soul. I'm singing, singing the sun above the horizon. Drumming, drumming, in rhythm with the gusting winds. I'm awaiting the fiercely tangled growth of spring.

Dreaming Seeds

Gardeners dream in seeds. All winter those potent points of life slumber, waiting expectantly for the first stirrings of spring. Now, as the days pass the spring equinox, the light luxuriously outstretching the dark, the gardener in me stirs. I read seed catalogues like pornography, with their promise of the perfect consummation of pleasure: the fragrant patch of basil, the unblemished bean leaves with slender pods unfurling between them, the shiny bodies of zucchini, the juicy cherries darkening on the bough.

I could spend days marking papers with squares and then filling them with the names of herbs and vegetables, and sketching a riot of flowers erupting between the intensively planted beds. I plot and scheme, seduced by the catalogue descriptions: Dragon carrots that ripen purple; Hidatsa beans with their stylishly speckled coats; the sweet flesh of Eel River melons that melt in the mouth. How could I not be titillated?

Today, in the barren brown of the first day of spring, I have no memory of picking aphids off potato leaves, mosquitoes swarming at sunset, or sun-reddened shoulders aching in the afternoon heat. Like the amnesia that soon envelops a newly crowned mother, I have forgotten the many seasons of labor pains that finally yielded food on the table. Instead, I remember True Siberian Kale melting in my mouth, and the taste of Purple Peruvian Potatoes mashed with garlic and unsalted butter. I recall the tang of nasturtium flowers with Forellenschloss lettuce, and herb dressing made from the herbs growing outside the back door: oregano, basil, sage, rosemary, and parsley.

I'm besotted. In the spring, I'm in love with the Earth again, a love so fresh and vital I have no room for caution, no carefully premeditated vow. I'm committed, yes; I'm blissfully, ignorantly devoted to this process of nurturing life.

You'd think I'd hesitate, even for a moment, after years of drought, hailstorms, floods, and desiccating winds. I know too much to make rash promises, to wed myself to this Earth.

Yet the love affair remains, like the unsullied love of teenagers still besotted in middle age. In truth, that's when my love affair began. I was 13, designing a vegetable garden in the back corner of our suburban yard. I stretched strings between sticks and planted straight rows of carrots, beets, spinach and turnips. I had globe artichokes, Swiss chard, and corn in orderly patches. Radishes and spring peas gave way to snap beans and winter squash. I watered every evening as the blaze of Ohio sun mellowed into gold, the light diffused in the humid haze of a breathless summer night. I loved weeding and caressing the seedlings, and then wading into the greenery as it reached my ankles, and later my knees and waist. My heart bloomed every time I approached the garden. I cherished that garden with the unfettered passion of first love, and the plants articulated their joy with luxurious growth.

In August, I reluctantly left the garden to work for a month at a summer camp in Michigan. I hated to leave my beloved garden. I begged my mother to let me pack two squash seedlings along with my cut-off jeans and tennis shoes. A gardener, too, she reluctantly agreed.

That summer my bedside reading was not Dickens or dime-store romances. I was reading *Peacock Manure and Marigolds* and Rodale's *Organic Gardening*. I had an insatiable desire to nurture those plants in every way possible. I was bonded with the garden by a love that had grown from the seeds of infatuation and ripened into a profound commitment.

The casually besotted seed catalogue reader becomes beloved partner in the garden when enough sweat has mingled with the Earth, enough tears have flooded with the rain, and enough love has been wrested from the daily tasks of weeding and hoeing and harvesting. The most profound love is cultivated in the mundane daily tasks of nurturing another's life.

Two Moons

This year a dear friend blessed me with an invitation to Passover Seder. I was deeply honored to join her extended family for this most sacred of holidays.

That evening we re-enacted the Hebrews' flight from slavery to freedom. I made that journey, in the intimacy of family, so that I would know where and what I had come from, because that knowledge shapes who I am now. We remember, with each sip of wine, with each taste of unleavened bread, how the Hebrews heard God's word and acted in complete faith. I trust God's word so fully that I leave *now*, placing the unbaked bread in my pack, allowing the desert heat to bake it flat as I cross that desolate land with my people. With each step, I am moving to freedom. I live this history in my own body, in the taste of this food, in the words of my ancestors forming in my mouth, in the sound of millennia-old chants ringing in my soul.

We read a section about Mitzrayim, "the narrow place," a point of land that separates two seas. What do I carry inside myself that separates me from the vast sea of God? What in me is like that spit of land?

We moved around the table, each one simply, honestly stating what separated us from Spirit. I named doubt, my uncertainty that I can accurately hear Spirit. I don't know if I would have stored the bread dough in my pack and abandoned my home in the middle of the night. Would I have listened? Would I have recognized Creator's voice amidst the cacophony of my own doubts?

The next morning I was thinking about the Last Supper, and I realized more fully than ever before that Jesus was sharing Passover Seder with his disciples. This was no ordinary meal. The Last Supper was the re-enactment of their people's flight from slavery to freedom. I understood more fully Jesus' revolutionary act of transforming the Passover symbols into his own truth. He intimately knew those symbols, so long held as touchstones by his people, and built from them a new truth. Did he prepare these words, or did they arise spontaneously from his profound understanding of his people's flight to freedom? Did he in that moment more fully understand his own journey, his own impending metamorphosis?

The unleavened bread, a remembrance of the Jews' trust in God's word, became Jesus' body. The wine, the remembrance of the Four Questions, became Christ's blood. Let these ancient symbols carry new, additional meaning. I have walked from slavery to freedom. Now I am walking away from the myth that life ends with death. With this bread, remember me. Remember that I am alive. With this wine, remember me. Remember that I live. Remember that you, too, can overcome death. My spirit, your spirit, will live beyond physical death. I am free from physical slavery, and I am also free from death. Let us walk across this desert and experience a new kind of freedom.

Perhaps this year the history awoke in me because the moon rose on the same weeknight Jesus was sharing Passover with his disciples. The same pearlescent light illuminated the robed men as Jesus bent to wash their feet. The same moon bathed my boys as their sleep-heavy heads rocked against the back seat of the car.

Today, new moon, is the beginning of the next lunar cycle, the celebration of Wesak, when the moon enters Taurus, the bull of fiercely grounded energy. In Buddhist tradition, the moon in Taurus marked three major events in Gautama Buddha's life: his birth, his enlightenment, and his death. Under this moon of effective action, Buddha planted the seeds of embodied wisdom.

According to esoteric traditions, on this full moon in Taurus, the wisdom of Buddha meets and melds with the love embodied in the Christ. The yang wisdom-mind mates with the yin-love of heart and soul. Together they give birth to – what?

At best, they give birth to my deepest, wisest, most loving self. My soul becomes manifest here on Earth, through the earth of my body. I welcome the strengths of each of these three traditions, sparking and blending one with the other, and creating something much greater than the sum of the parts.

I am not Jewish or Christian or Buddhist. On Wesak, I am the convergence of these streams, wisdom flowing into love and thereby dissolving illusion.

Passover gifts me with freedom from slavery. On Easter, I know freedom from death, and on Wesak I am freed from illusion. Free at last, free at last, free at last.

Meetings with Remarkable Trees

A 500-year-old oak, my favorite tree, stands in the wake of the Findhorn River, at the edge of a hayfield on Cawdor estate. At least three or four times a year during the time I lived in Scotland, I would ride my bike past the castle, famed setting of Shakespeare's *Macbeth*. The dirt lane headed northeast through a pine-tree plantation, a silent ecological desert almost completely bereft of birds and animals.

The lane crested a steep hill, and then I coasted into the hayfield, where a dozen ancient oaks lined the east edge of the field – all with craggy bark, their crevices deep enough to sink a fist almost to my elbow. Their limbs were arrested, twisted into arthritic gestures. Their trunks rose solidly for at least 70 feet, and their bases measured eight feet across.

I parked my bike and walked along the row, seeking my favorite among these centurions. My heart always quickened when I saw the blackened opening. I scrambled across a tangle of roots into the base of the tree and pushed myself up to sitting, my back resting against the charred innards of the tree. Never having met the groundskeeper, I always assumed the charring was intentional, perhaps a remedy for slow rot that had set into the heart of the tree. This wounding may have been from a chance crack deepened by insects and rodents, or the vagaries of time and weather. Whatever the source, the fire had feasted on the rotten wood and created a fertile womb.

I sat in the hollow belly of the oak, fingering the craggy bark at the entrance, listening to its strong-limbed boughs creak above me. Evening light tinted the freshly mown field with rusty gold. Pollen shimmered in a fluid haze above the shorn grass. In the muffled stillness, I inhaled the scent of grass pollen, dust, and summer sap.

I visited this wise elder many times over the years. On rainy days, I watched the drizzle from inside my leaf-lined nest. In the winter, snow highlighted the crags of the surrounding oaks, and the silent, furrowed field. In spring I almost heard the sap surging through the corky walls around me.

What farmer, I wondered, or gamekeeper or English laird pressed acorns into the soil, half a millennium ago? Who carried water from the river, first every day, then weekly, until the roots were deep enough to slake their own thirst? Who met under the branches for moonlit trysts? What children climbed the twisted boughs and sighted far-away lands from their crow's nest perch?

One hundred and fifty human generations have passed since these oaks began to grow. They have accrued time as layers of living wood. Over the years I developed a sense of a network of trees, like a communication grid that covered Britain and continued outward to encompass the whole of the planet. With deep sadness, I recognized that many links in the web were broken, as trees have died and not been replaced.

A couple of years later I visited Glastonbury, in part to visit Gog and Magog, the last remnants of a ceremonial corridor of oaks. On a winter afternoon I left the edges of the town to make my pilgrimage to visit these elders, survivors of more than 1,000 years. I walked the dirt farm lanes until I reached them. I could see craggy faces, with proboscis noses, in their profiles.

I sat with my back against one of the oaks, lingering as twilight deepened. Normally I do not see subtle colors, but in the wintry dusk I saw swirls of green and purple passing between these giants. I knew they were entangled by roots, time, and perhaps by love. Those colors bathed me as they swirled between these wise elders.

More than an accumulation of age, wisdom digests experience and weaves it into a tapestry of meaning. These trees have had centuries to accumulate their experiences of earth, moon and sky, and assimilate them through the furrowed structures of their bodies. Trees, in their fullest expression, mediate between heaven and earth. I count the oak at Cawdor Castle, Gog and Magog among the enlightened beings that have graced my life. These trees have transformed age into wisdom they freely share with those whose hearts are quiet enough to listen.

Snake Dreams

When I was a child, my brother brought home snakes from the nearby woods and kept them in a cardboard box. He taught me how to hold the garter snakes behind the head and allow them to coil around my freckled arms. I knew enough to respect the snakes; I was tentative, but not scared. My brother would keep them for a day or two, then release them in the woods. We'd watch as the snakes slithered like lightning into the dry leaves and disappeared into the welcoming woods.

On the winter solstice five years ago, I opened the back door of the house and discovered a small garter snake coiled next to the mat, basking in the pale mid-winter sun. I couldn't miss the snake's presence, so close to the door, nor the importance of the day – winter solstice, a time when most snakes were deep in hibernation.

Two weeks later I had the first of many dreams about snakes. In this dream, three viper snakes approached me. I ran, and they bit me in the back. I awoke with pain in the exact place where I had been bitten in the dream.

Snakes continued these nocturnal visits for more than a year. About 18 months later, I dreamt that I was digging a trench in a garden. The rectangular space was just big enough for me to lie in. I sat down in the hole. A green garden hose coiled next to me transformed into an enormous green snake with a woman's head. She had tousled blond hair and a mouthful of sharp, crooked teeth.

"Are you ready?" she asked lazily.

"Yes," I told her calmly.

She tipped her head back, then lunged, her teeth sinking into my back. I didn't flinch this time; I was ready for this kiss of transformation. I lay down in the hole, the exact size and shape of a grave, and slept within my dream. Again, I awoke feeling the "bite" in the exact spot in my back.

Last autumn, I walked into the root cellar and accidentally stepped on a snake. Thankfully, the garter snake was not injured. She slithered into the corner of the root cellar, looking for a relatively warm spot to overwinter. Traditionally Goddess figures draw their strength from the Earth, and snake is one of the most potent repositories of earth and kundalini power. Both the Virgin Mary and Avalokiteshvara often are depicted standing on snakes. They do not conquer the serpents; instead, they draw vitality from this potent source of life energy.

Kundalini power rises in the spine. In Hindi tradition the saints are depicted with a cobra snake erupting from their third eye, in the middle of the forehead. The snake slithers up the spine and blossoms in the third eye.

I'm still awaiting the full, volcanic eruption of kundalini power. Thankfully, the process for me has been a gentle boil, with chakras opening at different times. These energy centers have blasted open, one at a time, and then receded, with each chakra more open than before the blast. They have been permanently "stretched" by the extreme opening.

In the last month, as I've been writing a new book and re-awakening the creative power within me, I have dreamt of two snakes visiting me in the root cellar, which I understand to be my root chakra, the grounding of my vitality here on Earth. I know that spirit is stirring in me when snake slithers into my dreams.

Over time my fear of snake and its venom has softened. I continue to befriend snake, as much as one can "befriend" a volcano. I know its bite is intended to transform me. Snake slays what no longer serves me, opening the way for more vitality and creativity to erupt in my life. I sense that when I am able to welcome snake fully, she will slither up my spine and blossom in my forehead, and then I will be fully, completely awake.

Until then, I am satisfied with our nocturnal visits. I'm more comfortable with these dream encounters, just as I welcome the many garter snakes on the land. I have no desire to tame this wildness, only befriend it.

The Fifth Freedom

The summer after my sophomore year in college, I headed north on a Greyhound bus to work as a counselor at Farm and Wilderness, a Quaker camp nestled in the Green Mountains of central Vermont.

From the recruiting session that winter, I knew that Farm and Wilderness practiced what the founder Ken Webb called "The Fifth Freedom." Along with the four freedoms granted in the Bill of Rights, Ken added a fifth for campers, ". . . a freedom from clothes whenever no *rational* answer can be given to the question of why not?"

This freedom from clothes evolved during the first summer of the camp, later referred to as "the 1938 flood." On a rainy hike to a nearby pond, the boys realized they could arrive at the shelter with dry clothes if they stuffed them in their rucksacks and continued in their birthday suits. The method was so practical, so logical, that Ken Webb adopted the fifth freedom as a basic tenet of the camp.

During the first week of training, before the campers arrived, I spent the hour after lunch sunning on a dock that jutted out into the large lake rimmed with pine, maple and birch trees. Other counselors came to join me. Even though I told myself I was comfortable with my own and others' unclothed bodies, I still wasn't fully at ease. I made sure I met someone's eyes; I did not allow my gaze to stray. I wasn't going to view him or her as a pornographic image, a pop-up, two-dimensional starlet draped on a wilderness set.

Even though on a conscious level I was priding myself on my enlightened acceptance of nudity, I was still bucking my deeper conditioning: nudity and sexuality were one and the same, and certainly a full public display of nudity, and hence sexuality, was completely unacceptable.

When the campers arrived, I had two major responsibilities: a cabin of twelve-year-old girls; and swimming instruction at the waterfront with a team of five other counselors.

The main place where most of the campers exercised the fifth freedom was at the waterfront, and every morning I was there, teaching all levels of swimmers. I quickly grew to appreciate swimming unfettered by bathing suits – the smooth, unbroken flow of water over my body felt utterly natural. I soon began to wonder why I had ever worn a suit. As the summer progressed, the idea of wearing a heavy, wet suit – in or out of the water – seemed increasingly distasteful.

During the first week of camp, one of the younger kids, on scholarship from Brooklyn, NY, arrived at the waterfront with a camera. Meg, one of the waterfront staff, sidled up to her as she clicked pictures with her Kodak Instamatic.

"What are you doing, Keisha?"

"They're never gonna believe this in New York!" said Keisha.

By the end of the third week, Keisha arrived at the waterfront without her bathing suit. She jumped into the water with one arm flung overhead, the other gripping her nose, and she came up laughing and splashing her friends.

Meg casually walked over to the dock and caught Keisha's eye.

"Keisha," said Meg, "they're never gonna believe you in New York!"

Keisha blushed. We all laughed together.

By mid-summer, my pale, freckled skin had burned and baked into the closest I have ever come to an all-over tan. At the end of the fourth week, the camp hosted a special day for the arrival of campers for the second session. In addition, parents of the eight-week, full-season campers were welcome to visit for the day.

The waterfront staff met a few days before to discuss strategies for the open-swim period. In the past, one mother had withdrawn her child from the camp when she discovered the fifth freedom applied to adults as well as children. Every year the lifeguards had to grapple with whether or not to wear swim suits on parents' visiting day. Finally we agreed that each waterfront staff person would make her own decision, according to her own barometer of appropriateness.

Visiting day was a glorious, cloudless July day. I chose the floating raft about 100 yards from shore for my lifeguard post. I wore my whistle, and nothing else.

Soon the water was churning with swimmers of all ages. I was focused intently on the swimmers when a middle-aged woman hauled herself onto the raft.

"Are you someone official here?" she asked, staring up at me.

"Yes. I'm a lifeguard."

"Do you have a cabin?" she asked. "With campers?"

I could hear in the question her unspoken incredulity that a naked woman with a whistle around her neck could possibly have a position of authority.

"Yes. My cabin is Applegarth, with twelve-year-olds."

"Where are you from?" she asked.

"Ohio."

That final answer seemed to have clinched her confusion and discomfort. She slipped back into the water, and I did not see her for the rest of the day.

A week before the end of the summer, our cabin decided to hike eleven miles up the mountain to another part of the camp called Flying Cloud for a special naming ceremony. Flying Cloud, an all-boys' camp for ages 10 to 14, had no electricity or running water. The boys lived in tipis with their counselors and cooked all of their meals over open fires. Honoring Native American tradition, they had weekly sweat lodges as well as periodic naming ceremonies.

In many native tribes, a man or woman might have several names in a lifetime, each taken to honor a major transformation, a new responsibility, or a sacred revelation on their life path. The naming ceremonies at Flying Cloud were powerful gatherings that affirmed and celebrated the transformations the campers and counselors had undergone.

That night Flying Cloud was filled with visitors from other parts of the camp. The campers and counselors were serving bowls of stew from the large pots steaming over the open fires. I heard drum beats near the tiny sweat lodge perched next to the pond. I wanted to sweat before eating, and started down the hill toward the lodge.

"Judith!" called one of my friends, a counselor at Flying Cloud. His affinity for birds combined with his deep, loving heart, had earned him the name Kestrel-With-Open-Wings.

"Kestrel!" I said, hugging him warmly. "How are you?"

He smiled. "Good, good. Where are you going?"

"To the sweat lodge," I answered. "I'll see you at dinner!"

Kestrel continued walking up the hill, and I crawled into the sweat lodge just before the flap came down.

After several rounds of prayers, I crawled steaming from the lodge and plunged into the chilly, spring-fed pond. Only then did I realize that when Kestrel and I had met on the hill, neither one of us had been wearing clothes. Our greeting and physical contact were purely the loving gestures of two friends; our nakedness evoked no sexual spark.

In that moment, I understood the fifth freedom as far more than freedom from clothes. I was finally free of the burden of linking nudity with sexuality. I was free to enjoy my unfettered body without social mores or moralistic codes to bind me. I was free to enjoy the simple pleasures of skin meeting skin; skin meeting steam; and skin meeting cold, spring water without any cloth barriers to shield me from such pure delight.

Quaker traditions have long fostered respect for dissenting ideas and opinions. The Quakers seek truth, in all of its manifestations. Through that summer, my respect evolved to include both mental and physical realms. I discovered pleasure, far beyond sexual arousal, that engendered deep respect for my own and others' bodies.

Welfare

She was standing at the corner of SE 98th and Powell in Portland, Oregon. Her unzipped jacket was wrapped around her chest; the material no longer stretched to cover her pregnant belly.

A man stood next to her holding a hand-lettered sign, "Will work for food." This corner was a magnet for street people and laborers looking for a day's wages. Normally I drove through the intersection without a second glance, but on that Sunday morning my gaze snagged on that swollen belly, unprotected in the autumn drizzle.

I turned into a parking lot and turned off the engine. I had developed a personal policy of giving food but not money. I wouldn't hand someone a bag of heroin or methamphetamines, and I was not willing to hand them the money to support an addiction, either.

I climbed out of the car and walked over to the woman, now seated on the curb, hugging her swollen belly.

"Ma'am, do you need food?" I asked.

She stared up at me. "Yeah. We haven't eaten for three days."

"May I take you to the grocery store?"

She stared blankly for a moment; she seemed to have a hard time digesting the words.

She talked to the man carrying the sign, then turned back to me. "How far is the store?" she asked.

"About a mile-and-a-half."

She looked me squarely in the eye. I held her gaze. I sensed she was weighing my intentions against her hunger and distrust.

"All right," she said, nodding to the man. "My name is Mary, and this is my husband, Jack. I'll be right back," she said, giving her husband a quick hug.

As we drove to the store, Mary's story began to unfold. She and her husband had married a few months earlier and conceived soon after the wedding.

"We were living in California," she explained, "and everything was so expensive. We were looking for a place to move where we could get ahead, before the baby arrived."

A painting company in Portland, owned by an old family friend, offered her husband a job.

"We packed everything we could in the car and sold the rest." She stared out the window, watching the misty rain congeal on the glass. She took a deep breath and continued.

"We were coming north on I-5 when the car started to act up. Then it just quit. We didn't have enough money for a tow. We had saved $250, just enough to pay for food and gas to get to Portland.

"We had to leave the car and carry what we could in our arms. We hitchhiked to Portland and found the paint company."

She paused, tears pooling in her eyes. "In those three days, during our drive north, the paint company had gone out of business. We arrived in Portland with no car, no money, no job, and no place to stay."

"What did you do?" I asked.

"The people who owned the paint company said we could stay there, but after three days we didn't feel right, like we'd overstayed our welcome.

"So we went to Baloney Joe's for a night." Her face puckered. "That was *awful*. The beds were full of bugs. I couldn't sleep because my skin felt like it was crawling. We didn't stay there again."

"So where have you been staying?"

"Under the Burnside Bridge. That was actually cleaner than the flop house. I slept better there."

"When are you due?" I asked, imagining her trying to stay warm and dry under the bridge.

"Oh, I'm about five-and-a-half months pregnant. Baby's due in February."

We parked the car and walked into Albertson's. I pushed the cart, and Mary walked beside me.

I quickly realized she wasn't going to put anything in the cart, even though I could see the deep longing in her eyes as she surveyed the food.

"Do you need bread?" I asked.

She nodded.

"What kind?"

She pulled a loaf off the shelf. I put a second one beside it.

"How about fruit? Veggies?"

She put a couple of apples in the cart. I pulled a bag from the stand.

"Do you eat meat?"

"Doesn't everyone eat meat?" she asked, surprised.

I shrugged my shoulders.

She put a couple of packages of meat in the cart.

I was running through a list in my mind – what would she need? She clearly was not going to ask.

"How about toilet paper?" I asked. She nodded, and we wheeled the cart down another aisle.

We added a few more items, then went through the check-out line. I paid for the groceries, and we headed back to the car.

On the short drive back to the corner of 98th and Powell, Mary began to sob.

"I'm never going to look at street people the same way again."

When Mary got out of the car, I helped her unload the groceries and gave her one of my cards.

"You call me if you need help, OK?"

She nodded but would not look me in the eye.

"Promise?"

She nodded again.

I never heard from Mary or her husband again. I pray they found a job and an apartment before the baby arrived.

Mary got groceries that day, but I think I received a more valuable gift. I realized how close to the edge most of us live. A bad accident, a series of illnesses in the family, the death of a spouse, or the unexpected loss of a job could easily destroy someone laden with credit-card debt or stretched thin by a second mortgage. For most of us, our financial base is a house of cards, vulnerable to the shifting winds of fate.

"You know," said a friend recently, "I think welfare has created a whole generation of people who have absolutely no motivation to work."

"That may be true," I said, "but it's also created several generations of people who feel they no longer need to look out for their neighbor. Why should I help someone down the street when she could be on welfare?"

My friend knitted her brow. "Hmmm, I never thought of that," she said.

My brother lives in a farming community in central Ohio. A ninety-year-old neighbor down the road lost his wife more than 20 years ago. His next-door neighbors have brought him dinner every night since his wife's death. He never asked for help, and they never asked for permission. The neighbors simply cared for this elderly widower like one of their own.

When my neighbor in Portland had quadruple bypass surgery, I mowed his lawn weekly for a couple of months. I never asked if he needed help, and we never spoke of it afterward. This was my small, neighborly way of expressing my love and concern.

The welfare system has excused us from a vital truth: we are each other's keepers. Our most stable support, and our greatest security, is the web of family, friends and community.

Befriending Death

How often have I held concert with the silent, hooded oarsmen, who ferries the dead from this realm to others? No matter how often I have meditated on my own passing, preparing to release all that no longer serves me, I am uncomfortable with this neutral, faceless presence. When I step into the boat of the silent, hooded oarsmen, he offers no words of recognition, no touch of reassurance. Death is as neutral as water – a presence that flows into and through everything it touches.

We are all the clay molded by Death's constant presence. Who am I to think I might escape the oarsman's omnipresence? Who am I to think I might side-step this greatest defining dance?

In truth I've been dying since I was born. I've accumulated a comfortable heft of flesh and skill and experience, as if these substantial, physical things could shield me from their loss. Death tugs slowly but surely, as constant as gravity, on all I do in this daily round.

One of my dear friends is shrinking, her physical form devoured by the presence of cancer. As her physical body diminishes, her spirit shines more brightly. I see the fire in her eyes, the softness in her mouth. Time in the presence of death has sown compassion in her heart; the oarsman has that transformative effect on those who sit in that tiny wooden skiff, allowing the river currents to carry them to their destination.

But I'm not in that skiff, I defiantly tell myself. I don't have lumps or diseases or numbers on a chart to tell me that I am on that journey.

I draw a deep breath. More denial, more resistance. I've been sailing on this ship since the moment I drew breath.

And then last week the phone call came. My father has cancer. Such a small word has such a huge impact. The surgeon said the surgery "went well," and left the details for my mother and brother to share with my father. They chose to give my father a couple days of peace to recover from the surgery, and let the doctor deliver the news. What a horrid secret to keep, for the most compassionate of reasons.

"Well, at least I don't have any cancer," reported my surgery-weary father, triumph in his voice. He had vanquished his greatest fear – another paper dragon, those numbers and words on paper. Sadly, though, the reality of his death was stirring within him.

Cancer is the great awakener of this century, just as tuberculosis and the plague were awakeners of generations past. The frailty of the human body is the awakener, the stiff liquor of reality. I'm awake to the fact that those I love will be in this form for a limited amount of time.

I am offered the opportunity, if I want to take it as such, to revisit this silent presence, this guest who never really leaves the premises. I just manage to ignore death's presence, at my peril, for periods of time, when I am deeply engaged in the process of living.

Death reminds me that all I have is this moment, and this moment, and this moment. Anything else is immortalized only in memory. I have this second, this touch of the keyboard, this hum of the furnace. I have the silence of my mind and the fullness of my heart to buoy me.

In the end no one can divert me from this relationship with the oarsman who ferries me to my death. Sitting with him in silence, during my brief conscious forays in the boat, he offers no comfort, no explanation, no wisdom. The very neutrality of his presence forces me to turn within myself, to find the source of my own meaning and comfort.

And perhaps his method is precisely to take away all comfort, that great sedative that numbs me to my own situation. Let me sit in discomfort and know the reality of this moment, full on, no anesthesia, no thought of escape. The discomfort itself will help me stay awake to the reality of death, and the omnipresence of life.

He Is My Friend

When my friend, Phyllis, was a sprightly 82-year-old, she flew cross-country to attend my graduation from the Oregon College of Oriental Medicine.

Early on the morning of graduation, Phyllis called from New York's Laguardia Airport.

"My plane arrives at 11:15 a.m.," she said, her voice triumphant.

"Great!" I told her. "I'll be there."

I knew I would barely have enough time to pick up Phyllis, drop her bags at home, and then drive to the graduation site before the ceremony. Thankfully, Phyllis' plane arrived on time.

I watched Phyllis limp out of the jet way and knew her left hip was in terrible pain. When I asked how she was feeling, Phyllis dismissed me with a wave of her hand. Without a protest, though, she accepted my offer to push her in a wheelchair to the baggage claim area.

As we waited for her small tote bag at the luggage carousel, I asked about her other bags.

"They're in New York," she said simply.

"New York?"

"Yes, New York."

"What are they doing *there*?"

"Last night I was talking with my friends Ed and Marilyn, who drove me from Massachusetts to New York for a friend's birthday party. They told me under no circumstances was I to fly to Portland. They said I simply wasn't strong enough."

Phyllis rolled her eyes.

"I tried to tell them about when I was living in the Middle East, and some friends and I were traveling across the desert in a car. A few miles after leaving the last town, we saw a man on the road.

"We stopped to offer him a ride, but he was walking in the opposite direction. He had walked many miles, alone, from a distant village.

"'Where are you going?' we asked him.

"'My friend is leaving," he explained, 'to move to another country. I had to come see him.'

"'But surely your friend wouldn't expect you to walk . . . .'

"'But he is my *friend*,' the man repeated. 'I had to come see him.'

"I was trying to explain to Ed and Marilyn that you were my *friend*." Phyllis threw up her hands and shook her head. "They just didn't get it."

"So what happened to the bags?"

"Ed and Marilyn locked them in their car before they went to bed. When I got up at 5 a.m., they were asleep. I called a taxi and went to the airport." Her eyes twinkled. "I still had my wallet. And at the airport I bought one of those senior passes, you know, $100 for each leg of the journey. I used two passes to get here."

We arrived at the house, and I went inside to gather my things before leaving for the graduation ceremony. Phyllis followed me into the bedroom.

"So," she said, "what am I wearing?"

I pulled out a free-flowing dress that draped artfully over her self-described E.T. body, and found a pair of shoes that fit.

On the highway, driving cross-town, Phyllis apologized profusely for not having her video camera.

"I *promised* I would tape the graduation," she said, "and my camera is locked in the trunk of that car in Manhattan."

Phyllis grew quiet, and I knew she was focusing her mind on what she wanted. "I promised . . . . I promised . . . ." she muttered.

When we arrived at the graduation site, I made sure Phyllis was settled in the front row before joining my classmates in a back room. A few minutes before the ceremony was to begin, I sneaked back into the auditorium to check on Phyllis.

"Judith!" she yelled when she caught sight of me. She waved a shiny video camera in her right hand.

"Where did you get *that*?" I asked.

"Oh, the woman next to me was telling me how she had just bought this video camera and had no idea how to use it. She asked me to film the whole graduation. See, I told you I'd make a tape for you!"

She pressed her eye against the viewfinder and continued to scan the stage, preparing for her production.

I smiled and returned to the waiting room with my classmates. For me, the graduation ceremony was incidental. Phyllis was the real celebration. Like the man walking across the desert, magnetized by love for his friend, Phyllis had come. She drew to her all that was luminous, outrageous and whole. Like the man awaiting his friend at the edge of the sands, I received Phyllis. Her presence anointed me, like rain in the desert, moistening every crevice in my soul.

From the Inside Out

Who do I long for in my darkest, loneliest moments?

I think of all of the soldiers whose final word, as they lay in their own crimson life source, was, "Mother."

They came in bathed in their mother's blood – wet, shining, bloody with joy as they reached for first breath.

There on the battlefield, faces turned to the endless blue, again bathed with blood, reaching for last breath – the soldiers called for mother.

Mother is our entry and our longed-for exit.

My own mother cleaved her flesh into three – a daughter, a son, and another daughter. The river of ancestors ran through her, eddying just long enough for us to catch our breath.

Deep in my cells, I know my mother's arms, the texture of her skin, the tang of her sweat. I know her, literally, from the inside out.

Years ago, shortly after my sister's death, I met my mother at the airport. As she walked through the gateway into my waiting arms, tears welled in my eyes. Before I touched my mother, I smelled her – the salty scent of "honest sweat," as she called it, unadulterated by perfumes. This was the scent of a woman damp from digging in the garden, hot from pulling weeds, moist from the work of chasing children and managing a home.

Through this scent, I know my mother from the inside out.

I know her sound as well. I could find her in a crowd with my eyes closed. There's that nuance, the pause, before, "Well . . . ." which means, "I'm thinking. I'm giving you that Midwestern modicum of courteous restraint. I'm listening to your opinion, even though I don't agree."

I know my mother by touch, as well. The skin is thinning now, but still smooth, summer-brown from the biceps down, sun-kissed from years of tucking plants in the soil, hauling buckets, and tending the gardens she loves.

I know my mother by the bent of her mind. Christened "mettlesome Mattie" as a child for her insatiable curiosity, she is still driven by that restless pursuit of knowledge. Her roving brain can search and collate historical data, the shreds of lives and towns gone by, and make a tapestry of meaning from those details.

I know my mother by her spirit, for her indomitable will to *do*. She was shaped by World War II, a member of "The Silent Generation" who learned to endure, to make do, to bear without complaint. She came of age in a generation devoted to productivity, to making things right, to solving the world's great problems with technology. From Depression to dominion they rose, the rulers of the free world.

When that ancestral river entered my own veins, I had a completely new understanding of "mother." I felt those babies, a moving sea of bumps and kicks within me, yet also entirely their own beings. I also knew them from the inside out.

When they emerged in the world, we began our journey of separation and individuation. From shared heartbeat we moved to shared bed, then shared home. Someday soon we will graduate to shared community and then world.

I watch the boys now, their sprouting limbs swatting hard at baseballs, running around the sandy baseball diamond, and I see they are shaping their own bodies, their own worlds.

Still, when they cross the home plate, a look of triumph blossoming on their flushed cheeks, they wait at the fence outside the dugout to catch my eye, to grin and give me a "thumbs up" salute.

The umbilical cords have long since been cut, but heart threads still gently bind us.

So we have memories, a history compiled like sedimentary rock from the accumulation of daily sharing: a word, a touch, a salty scent. All of those shared events – from mundane to momentous – create the solid rock of relationship that I call "mother."

That's the infallible support most of us turn to as we slip from this flesh – all of the small, often overlooked moments that gradually congeal to become "mother," the center of gravity, the defining pull of one's life.

Food

Recently I awoke from a dream sweating from the effort of talking to a group of farmers in a field. In my waking life, I was recovering from laryngitis. In the dream, though, I was standing in a plowed field with my family and a group of about 20 farmers. They were debating the use of Round Up and other chemicals on their crops.

As the meeting neared its end, I began to shout. "The issue is about *quality*, not quantity of food." The farmers looked at me, perplexed.

I awoke thinking of *The Omnivore's Dilemma*, an expose of how over-production of corn has affected the US food supply for the last century. In the 19th and early 20th centuries, farmers increased the value of their corn crop by turning it into whiskey. Today cheaply produced corn drives a host of poor food decisions, including feeding corn to cows (who are meant to eat grass), which contributes to a whole range of bovine diseases including deadly *E. coli* overgrowth. Corn is also used to make cheap sweeteners, such as high-fructose corn syrup and dextrose. Corn has infiltrated nearly every crevice of our food supply.

Monsanto, the chemical siren who supplies the poisons intended to protect and prod plants into full production, has become a wicked step-mother in the food supply. Recent research presented by Dr. Huber, a retired soil biologist from Purdue University, reveals that Roundup not only kills weeds but also destroys the microorganisms in the soil that allow rootlets to absorb nutrients. Over time, Roundup applications produce super-bacteria that infect every aspect of the food supply, including us.

What does this have to do with me, with us? Everything, from our breakfast to our dinner to our annual check-ups. Finally, after years of denial, the U.S. government is acknowledging that the skyrocketing rates of cancer are directly linked with chemical exposures. We are what we eat: what the animals we consume have eaten; what the fish we eat have swum in; and what the plants we ingest have been bathed in. We are the sum of all of the exposures of every aspect of our food supply.

So here's the garden I choose to eat from: local farmers who have raised plants and animals with sun and rain, manure and ash, love and consciousness. I choose to vote with my hard-earned dollars for organically grown food raised in my neighborhood, *not* something trucked thousands of miles from California or Mexico, or flown from New Zealand. I want something infinitely more radical, and infinitely simpler: local, organic food. I want greens ripened in March cold frames, cherries harvested under Fourth of July fireworks, garlic pulled from the August-baked soil, and apples blushing in the warm September sun. I want food metamorphosed from the soil I walk on.

I'm hungry for quality, not quantity of food. I used to joke about gourmet restaurants serving homeopathic doses of food. I've grown used to the lure of cheap, abundant, nutrient-starved food. My body needs more of this denatured food to survive. Eating densely nutrient-rich food, though, I need so much less to thrive.

Thich Nhat Hanh also reminds me that *how* I eat influences the benefit I receive from the food. I look at my family sitting at the table. We offer thanks for the day. Usually the conversation devolves into a stream-of-consciousness potpourri of lines from movies mixed with super hero fantasies and playground antics.

Thich Nhat Hanh reminds me to look down at the plate and allow the food to become real. "This food reveals our connection with the Earth," says Hanh. "Each bite contains the life of the sun and the earth. The extent to which our food reveals itself depends on us. We can see and taste the whole universe in a piece of bread!"

Eating and tasting, I wake up to the nourishment at the table. I am fed by my family; I am nourished by my food. I'm angling for quality rather than quantity. My food choices will either weave me into the web of life or tear it asunder.

Field of Dreams

I'm not a flag-waving patriot, brandishing hot dogs, apple pie, and a Chevy pickup, but baseball stirs in me a sense of what is good and right in our topsy-turvy culture.

This spring, my boys joined a Little League baseball team for the first time. Early on opening day, pick-up trucks decorated with streamers and loaded with uniformed boys and girls paraded through the city streets and then climbed the hill to the mesa where backstops lean against a panorama of craggy, snow-covered peaks.

A line of more than two dozen trucks snaked up the hill, horns blaring, balloons streaming, kids shouting. The youngest tumbled out first, four- and five-year-olds swarming like restless gnats in their micro-sized cleats. With coaxing, they began the stream of players surging toward the fields – progressively older boys and girls, jerseys and hats proclaiming their allegiance with a major-league team. The Little League teams ran out on the field, one after the other, and stood at attention as we sang the national anthem.

We listened as one of the boys recited the Little League oath: "I trust in God. I love my country, and I will respect its laws. I will play fair and strive to win, but win or lose, I will always do my best."

Tears streaked my face. I didn't expect this invocation of character, of developing moral as well as physical sinew. The ceremony caught me off guard. These kids were rehearsing for the big leagues, with the same pageantry on opening day. The parents and coaches were summoning greatness from these fledgling players.

And so began a season – of perfect hits, spectacular catches, heroic throws, and breath-taking saves – all played on a field of dreams on that chilly, windy morning as the boys and girls stood in their untried, unstained uniforms.

Within minutes, with the throwing of the first pitch, those dreams gathered the grit and dust of reality – learning to deal with disappointment as the umpire called the third strike, struggling with humiliation as the fly ball bounced off the glove, cringing as the runner on third plowed into the waiting catcher clutching the would-be home-run ball. Quickly the dusty field swallowed those dreams and transformed them into something bigger: lessons in defeat and stubborn resurrection that would serve these girls and boys for a lifetime.

After living outside the United States for several years, I came home for reasons that are invisible from a distance, screened by our government's swaggering international stance. I returned because of a people who value dreams, who have the courage to seed them in their children, and who are willing to create an environment for them to fail, falter, and finally fly. Little League, big dreams, small bodies, large hearts – this is the stuff that can make our nation great.

No Regrets

After placing last in the national championships, Apollo Ohno's father took him to a remote cabin and left him alone for several days. "You take this time to decide," said his father, Yuki. "Are you going to compete or not? Either give yourself fully, or stop. You choose."

Apolo was being asked to decide how he wanted to direct his passion and energy. He chose to dedicate himself fully to short track speed skating. He chose to live without regrets.

Three years ago, when my brother, Tom, knew my father would soon be passing, he sold his business so he could have more time with our father.

"I realized time was passing," said Tom, "time I wouldn't be able to get back, and I had things I wanted to do with Dad."

Tom joined my father for weekly model-airplane-flying sessions in a grassy meadow between Ohio cornfields. "At first I was going for Dad," said Tom, "but after a while, I realized I was getting back much more than I was giving. Dad's flying buddies became my friends, too."

Already an expert woodworker, Tom began building model airplanes with my dad. Tom's barn that once housed his staircase construction company metamorphosed into a model-airplane-building shop. He bought a trailer to haul the planes and other equipment. Tom traveled with Dad to Indiana each summer for the national model-airplane-flying championships.

Last July, Tom packed his trailer with one of his favorite planes and an engine he and my dad had bought a couple of years earlier but had never used.

When the event began, Tom struggled to start the engine. Finally, the dormant engine sputtered to life, and Tom maneuvered the airplane into the sky.

Dad watched as the plane soared for more than 45 minutes, winning the event by several minutes.

I have a photo of my father, Tom, and his son, Bill on the national championship field with the plane in front of them and Tom cradling the trophy.

"I did that for Dad," said Tom, smiling at the photo. "I wanted him to have the pleasure of seeing that engine flying."

Tom also arranged to have a master model builder complete and then fly Dad's last model airplane. We have a video of the plane taking off, always a breathless moment for a model-plane builder, as hundreds of hours and years of work either soar into the sky or smash into pieces on the ground. In the video, Dad's tight mouth eases into a grin as he watches the plane sail into the sky.

In September, just four months before Dad's passing, Tom finished Dad's remote-control boat and invited him to the farm to sail the boat on the pond. Dad stood on the bank of the pond, deeply satisfied as he steered the boat across the water.

A couple of months before he passed, Dad began a new model airplane. Tom joined him in the construction as Dad's hands lost their dexterity and he fumbled with the tiny parts.

The day Dad went into Hospice, a package arrived with two gallons of lacquer paint to finish the airplane. I looked at those paint cans, a lifetime supply for a model builder, and knew Dad had ordered them for Tom. Dad was making sure Tom would have all he needed to continue with his friends – *their* friends – in making and flying model airplanes.

When Tom picked me up at the airport, just 12 hours before our dad's passing, I asked how he was doing.

Tears gathered at the corners of his eyes. "I have no regrets," he said evenly. He shared all of the events of the previous year, fishing in the afternoons at the farm, flying planes with Dad, winning the national championship in Indiana.

"All of that was for Dad, not me. I made sure he finished everything on his bucket list. I thought I was doing all those things for him, but now I realize I got so much more back. I have no regrets."

This Father's Day I have memories to nurture, and deep gratitude for my brother, who made choices so that both he and my father could live, and die, with no regrets.

SUMMER

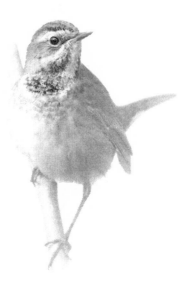

Summer Fullness

Today I am full of rock and flower, cloud and hail. I'm the elements thrusting up as pine tree, as luxuriant mountain bluebell, as electrified Indian paintbrush. I've ingested silica, mica, sandstone and granite to create a palette of colors unequaled in any museum – buttercup yellow, magenta paintbrush, violet larkspur, dainty pink wild geranium.

Walking at 12,500 feet in Yankee Boy Basin, I can feel how this land has a fingernail hold on summer. Sheets of snow, dusted with windblown red Utah dirt, still hover above streams and cling to shadowy crevasses. The earth is just bare, the sun kissing the scree slopes and thin-skinned land, catalyzing an eruption of miniature flowers. Larkspur bobs three inches above the ground, Indian paintbrush sways at two inches, and Saxifrage snuggles against the rock, with a showy spray of flowers atop a moss-like mat of green leaves.

Hunkering down, these alpine survivors dig roots into the scattered rock. They shoulder hail and snow, even at this fullest moment of summer.

A pika squeaks and then scurries across the scree slope. A chipmunk, also more compact than I've seen on the lower, forested slope, bullets across the path to a more distant perch.

Compact, essential, vibrant with life – this is the compressed life cycle of an alpine ecosystem. I sense the urgency of this miniaturized community as thunder booms in the basin, reverberating through my body. Rain and hail pelt my bare legs; I'm grateful for my hat and waterproof jacket. The storm catalyzes movement. Even with an injured knee, I move swiftly down the slope.

The storm passes, leaving a sheen of rain on the rocks. The wildflowers are even more dazzling with their thirst slaked by the icy rain.

The distant slope of Stony Mountain now glistens emerald green. The world is renewed with this Eucharist of the elements.

I reach again and again for my camera, hoping to record this moment on film. I know, though, that I'm grasping at clouds. Even in its fullness, this mountain Valhalla is preparing for its transfiguration. The marmot that surfaces briefly among a sea of rocks looks fat and sleek. Already she is preparing for winter. Some of the first spring wildflowers have already set seed and released them to the gusty winds.

I want to savor this riot of color and sensuous abundance. The harder I grasp, though, the more I crush its succulent splendor.

So let me savor this summer peak, feeling the sap rising in my bones and unfurling as ephemeral breezes on my sun-bared skin. Help me sense the vitality of elements coalescing in these magnificent forms. Let me hold this fullness lightly.

Like the Taoists, I know that the greatest expression of yang holds the seed of yin within it. The supreme expression of life, this summer revolution of elemental form and color, holds the seed of deepest winter. Even within growth, and in the richest expression of creativity, I catch the scent of sour decay. At birth, we begin our careening course toward death.

For now, may I enjoy the elements in my own body, surging at their highest tide – my own form moving with ease through this rock-boned, flower-spangled landscape. May I enjoy, savoring the fullness, knowing I am casting seed to survive my own winter of darkness, my own season of age, death and new becoming.

River of Ancestors

I swam here through a river of ancestors, a stream that flows back to the first spark of life. Those ancestors have nurtured me on many levels, providing the physical substrate that is my body, and the cellular structure of my soul.

For years I wooed that river of ancestors, aching for its waters to flow through and beyond me, carrying life into another generation. I longed for solid flesh, not night-spun dreams, to warm my soul.

The night my great Aunt Loey died, and before I knew of her passing, I dreamed three generations of sisters (my mother and her sister Muffy; my grandmother Gladys and her sister Loey; my sister Ruth and I) were traveling in an old roadster across the Midwest. We stopped at a motel for the night. While I bathed in a tub at the back of the property, in the open air with soft evening breezes stirring the trees, a chamber maid came to chat with me.

"So," she said, "you're tourists."

"No," I told her decisively. "We are travelers with a purpose."

My family is a weaving of Amazons, a tapestry of strong women who have given their lives to something greater than themselves. In my thirties, though, I was aware that three of those women were childless, some by design, others by default.

"Don't wait too long," my aunt Loey warned me a couple of weeks after I graduated from college.

"For what?" I asked, although I knew her meaning.

"To find a man and get married. Don't wait like I did."

I remember Great Aunt Eleanor laughing about sneaking into her older sisters' closets and snitching chocolates carefully hidden in their corsets. Her older sisters certainly had gift-bearing suitors. I know Loey loved at least a couple of men, but her family didn't approve of one, and the other was too short, so she dismissed them.

Most of my adult life I have lived alone, moving amidst crowds and families and couples like an unmatched mitten. Mostly I have been comfortable with my singular presence in the world, but at times I have struggled with loneliness. I wonder if Loey, too, was buffeted by her solitude?

My mother and her generation considered Loey their second mother. Perhaps she unleashed all of her maternal loving on her nieces and nephews. Maybe Loey mated with the world instead of with a man. But Loey, did you ever long for flesh and blood? Did you ever shed tears for the children who never flowered in your womb? Did you ever cry for arms to encircle your own, creating islands of refuge in your aloneness?

Maybe you lived beyond all these things and learned not to regret. Maybe you created a house of your own loving. Were you a virgin when they returned you to the soil, your blossom still unfurled in your passing? How did you survive without loving?

I'm too full of soil, too rich with worms and buried secrets to live my life without physical loving. I chose to bring forth the fruit of my womb and create a family in my life. No immaculate conception, but rather a flesh and blood celebration of living. I sent my root deep into the earth, accepted the gifts of sun and wind and rain, bit down on the bitter elements of earth, and passed the seed of loving to my offspring, that they might pass the gift to others.

Thank you, ancestors, for the gift of love that sparked my life. I honor your courage in allowing life to flow through you, for flesh to root and grow and seed within you, to be released into the world. Thanks for the gifts that live in me: a love of soil and beauty, of words and travel, of sunsets and bird tracks in wet sand. I carry farmer, herbalist, healer, physician, musician, writer, scholar, artist in my blood. I will pass them on. To seven generations, I will pass them on.

The Heart of India

When I was preparing to leave Scotland for India, at least half a dozen people in the community where I lived approached me to share *their* experiences of India. The majority spoke of stolen suitcases, swindled money, illness, filthy toilets, and assaulted women. By the time I arrived in India, I was so frightened I could not sleep. I rode twelve hours on the bus without getting out to pee; I wasn't ready to face the toilets yet. I arrived at my destination exhausted from the physical tension. I lived in southern India for almost five months. Only in the last month did I finally relax and enjoy my sojourn.

Toward the end of my stay I traveled to Tiruvannamalai, a temple town at the base of Arunchela, a sacred mountain regarded by the Hindus as the navel of the universe. I spent three days in Sriraman Ashram, a small community dedicated to the teachings of Ramana Maharshi, a great teacher who lived during the first half of the twentieth century.

When I entered the hall for the afternoon *puja* before the tomb of Ramana Maharshi, I had the sense of a community focused on perpetuating the memory of a ghost. After the ceremony, I walked across the courtyard and climbed a short way up the mountain to watch the sunset.

When I returned along the path, I was not surprised to see a saffron-robed old man approaching in the evening mist. What was unusual, though, was his warm smile and peaceful nod.

"Good Evenick," he said. "I recognize you from the meditation hall. You sit for a long time." He nodded approvingly. "Ver-r-r-ry good."

We walked for a while together along the path. He pointed to himself and said, "Satyananda." I rolled the name in my mouth and then clumsily spilled it out. He smiled and pointed to me.

"Judith," I told him.

He began to tell me stories about his life here at the foot of Arunchela, of his time as Ramana Maharshi's personal attendant, the most joyful years of his life. After his beloved master's death, Satyananda took a vow of silence for nearly 20 years. Soon after his decision to speak again he moved out of the ashram and into his own small hut.

"Why did you go?" I asked.

"Too much fighting, too much politics. I was tired of it, so I came to live here," he said, pointing down the path. "Come, see where I live. I will show you. And I show you my photo album."

I was a bit uncertain about following the old man. I'd heard stories about licentious sadhus (renunciates) who were less than virtuous in their dealings with lone women – but he seemed kind-hearted, so I decided to follow.

His tiny two-room mud brick house was mostly bare except for pictures of Ramana Maharshi. The altar, though, was crammed with cards and memorabilia from people who had visited him from all over the world. He pulled a well-worn photo album from beneath his simple cot and placed it before me, nodding. Among the carefully pasted pages were many pictures of Ramana Maharshi, clothed only in a loincloth, his great height accentuated by the tiny attendant – Satyananda – who appeared in each picture, as persistent as a shadow.

When I stood to leave, I felt my heart fly open, ignited by the simplicity of this man's devotion. He clasped my elbows and pressed his cheek against mine and then leaned back to hold my gaze for a few moments.

Before I left he invited me to tea in the morning, and I promised to return at 10:30 a.m.

The next morning I stopped to buy bananas at a local stand to give to Satyananda and then walked along the dirt road that led to his tiny house. Satyananda gratefully accepted the bananas and placed them amidst the clutter on the altar.

"Puja, puja," he said, smiling. I sat quietly on the floor while he patiently opened containers from the pile of cookie tins that filled one corner of the room. He withdrew tea and powdered milk and then boiled water on his single gas ring. While the water heated, he carefully arranged a handful of nuts and cookies on a small plate. My chest ached as my heart opened wide – for the first time, I realized, since arriving in India. We sat in silence, listening to the birds chirping in the trees outside until the water hissed in the pot. He prepared the tea and set the single cup before me. I looked up, surprised – nothing for him? He swiveled his head and motioned for me to drink, so I slowly sipped the sweet, milky tea and ate the nuts and cookies on my plate. When I finished we sat quietly for a few more minutes until I nodded my head to tell him I must go.

"Yes," he said, nodding, "lunchtime at the ashram. But I not eat today. Full moon. Beginning of Tamil month, and Friday," explained Satyananda, holding up three fingers. "Very important. Today I walk around Arunchela with visiting sadhu and man from France living here with us. You are welcome to come," he said simply. "Meet us here at 3:30. Long walk – 13 miles. We maybe go to temple afterwards."

I thanked him, moved by his invitation, and promised to come. I wouldn't have missed the chance to walk around the mountain under the full moon for anything.

At 3:30 p.m. the sun was still hot as we turned off the dirt path and onto the bitumen road in front of the ashram. We joined a swell of villagers making their way from the center of Tiruvannamalai back to their villages. They stopped in ones and twos at the small Shiva temples that peppered the base of the mountain to "make puja," a ritual of purification performed by the resident holy man. After about an hour we turned to the right along a dirt road that skirted the western side of the mountain.

By the time we reached the town of Tiruvannamalai on the far side of Arunchela, the streets had darkened, and the moon hung just above the top of the mountain. After a simple dinner of dosas at a local restaurant and shopping for vegetables, we made our way to the temple.

The temple was thrumming with activity. Satyananda was in his element. The priests bowed respectfully and smiled as he passed. He obviously was a well-known and much loved figure. We sat for a while on some steps, eating milk candy and sharing it with the children and beggars thronging the area.

Eventually we moved through the temple and into the dark streets, walking the last miles around the mountain and back to

Sriraman Ashram. At the gate I waved good-bye to the others and returned alone to my simple room.

"Thank you, Creator," I murmured as I undressed and pulled the single sheet over me. Until the last few days India had felt like an alien land. The time in the ashram, though, had awakened some sleepy, half-forgotten memory: if not of this specific place, then perhaps of this way of life, of simple devotion and one-pointed focus on inner development. I had found the loving heart in the stern disciplinarian of Mother India.

Birdie

One summer, I worked with my dear friend, Phoebe, to create Findhorn U.S.A., a resource center in North America for the community in Scotland. One morning in late July, before the sun had reached its mid-day swelter, Phoebe discovered a baby sparrow that had fallen from its nest.

Phoebe filled a hot water bottle, covered it with a towel, and placed the tiny bird in the soft folds of cloth. She called the Audubon Society for direction. They suggested hourly feedings but were not very encouraging about the bird's survival.

That night, Phoebe woke every hour to feed the sparrow. A day passed, and then another. The baby was passing, moment by moment, beyond the critical zone. "Birdie," as we named the sparrow, developed a loud squawk to demand food or general attention.

One small miracle followed another until one morning, we placed Birdie on the back porch and watched him lift on stuttering wings. After a few test flights, Birdie soared around the yard and landed on the back fence.

We watched anxiously throughout the day to see whether Birdie would return to his box-nest. He roosted in the box a few times, but each visit was shorter until finally, he abandoned his "nest" altogether.

Although I had always heard that a baby animal touched by humans would be rejected by others of its kind, Phoebe and I witnessed an extraordinary outpouring of support for Birdie. Soon after sunrise we would hear Birdie's unmistakable "CHEEP." Sitting at the breakfast nook we watched a procession of birds, of all species and sexes, line up on the back fence to feed Birdie. Far from being rejected, Birdie became the prodigal son of the neighborhood birds. Birdie was a living demonstration of the strength of community, and an inspiration for the resource center Phoebe and I were creating.

Five years passed. The summer before entering naturopathic medical school, I lived for two months in Ohio with my parents, a welcome sojourn as I moved from east to west coast. I developed a rhythm of working during the day and walking in the evenings when the heat and humidity began to abate.

During one such walk, I heard squawking in a neighbor's yard. As I moved closer, I saw two mourning doves sitting on the lowest branch of a tree, their necks extended toward a fledgling flopping on the ground. By the time I reached the grassy lawn, the fledgling lay face down, with its wings splayed on either side.

I looked up at the parents, wondering if they were capable of airlifting their almost-grown fledgling. They squawked and flapped but made no attempt to assist their offspring.

I headed home to find a box to carry the bird. I decided that if the juvenile mourning dove was still there when I returned, I was meant to shelter it until it could fly on its own.

I gently scooped up the bird and placed it in the box. At home I added a bowl of water and bird seed. As the sun sank below the horizon, I debated whether to leave the bird on the porch, in the cool evening air, or to bring it into the stifling house, still radiant with 100-degree summer heat. I decided to leave the bird outside.

I placed a wire mesh on top, to keep out predators, and covered the box with a towel. This "baby" was almost fully grown, so I assumed it would not need hourly feedings.

I hesitated one more time, wondering whether to bring the bird inside. The dove had recovered from its catatonic state and was chirping quietly and moving around in the box. I finally decided the bird would be more comfortable outside.

I awoke early in the morning and immediately went to check on the mourning dove. I lifted the towel and was shocked to discover the dove lying limp, its twisted neck drowned in the water dish.

Did the bird fall into the water, I wondered, or was this suicide? In that moment I realized the fledgling was accustomed to the constant touch of its parents. That night was likely the first it had ever spent alone. Perhaps this adolescent bird had died of loneliness.

I realized the dove might have survived if I had brought the box inside. More than food or water, the fledgling needed love to survive. In its passing the bird offered me one of the greatest lessons of my medical career: food, water, and shelter alone will not heal. All therapies are impotent without the greatest medicine, which is love.

Wild

Walking into Mount Sneffels Wilderness, I ask myself why I am so drawn to wild places. Trekking up the steep path, I know the challenges of moving and living in such places. Sliding down the path in a thunderous downpour, my boots finding no purchase in the slick mud, I also know that wildness cannot be romanticized. Wilderness requires much more awareness and much more effort than my sedentary, domesticated life. I lose comfort; I gain aliveness.

When I say "wild," most people think "out of control," "feral" – something once tamed that has gone awry, like a rabid dog.

For me, though, wild means pristine, still rooted in native habitat and governed by natural rhythms.

Walking along the path, I am struck by the mélange of colors – brilliant pink Indian paintbrush nestled amongst indigo larkspur, cow parsnip, and golden blanket flowers. My gardening friend would shudder at this riotous mix of colors. Here, though, these succulent, storm-drenched plants harmonize a cacophony of color.

As I walk through old-growth forest, I wonder what I would be like if I allowed my wild roots to blossom and set fruit. I don't mean allowing myself to become feral, with my domesticated branches tangling and going to seed. I mean bringing up strength from my deepest, wildest roots.

Like the aspen, I'd be relaxing into the soil, reaching up for light in the canopy, and giving rise to new seedlings at the far edges of my roots. I would be enmeshed in a community of aspen, connected by subterranean roots that make these trees the largest living organisms on the planet.

Like a grouse with a wounded wing, I would turn inward for healing. When injured, the grouse does not push herself to shop for groceries or attend a board meeting. She understands the importance of drawing inward and giving herself fully to healing.

Like the chipmunks, I would move with the sunlight and take cover when thunder boomed in the valley and reverberated among the surrounding stony peaks. I'd move quickly when I perceived danger; I'd sit in attentive stillness when I was at peace, with no threat to attend to. I would cultivate my energy carefully and spend it wisely.

Joy, I've learned, is the exception. Late one spring afternoon in Mesa Verde, with snow dusting the craggy cliffs, I watched crows soaring in the updrafts. They called lazily to one another. I cast a few calls into the stillness and listened for a ripple of sound in response. We conversed a bit, the crows and I. Two crows approached the rim of the valley, careening toward an overhanging pine tree. I laughed out loud as one of the crows rolled and made a loop-the-loop before landing lightly on the branch.

Expressing joy, I understand, is not frivolous, but rather a nutrient as vital as food and water.

True wildness bypasses reckless abandon in favor of honoring natural rhythms, something the Taoists and most indigenous people have known and practiced for millennia. Wildness means honoring and nurturing innate wisdom, focus, and balance instead of abandoning my essence to chaos. I might forsake recklessness as I surrender to wildness, but what I receive in compensation is enormous – the support of an immeasurable universal flow that buoys and directs me, that informs and enlivens everything it touches.

So let me ease my feet into the waters, breathe deeply, and release myself into the current. Traveling this river does not excuse me from attentiveness; this is no "free ride." On the contrary, riding the rapids and negotiating eddies requires a wakefulness I've forsaken in my river-bank life. Moving with the currents will require more attentiveness, not less.

What do I gain in this surrender? I look into the alert eyes of my wild companions and discover my own wakefulness. I gain buoyancy as I enter an infinite stream much larger than any flow of my own making. As I soar, calling to my companions across the valley, I allow joy to roll and twirl me into astonishing acrobatics.

Wild, not reckless; focused, not feral. I give up my cozy seat and my climate-controlled ease for something less comfortable, and supremely more satisfying: buoyancy, harmony, wakefulness, joy.

Nuclear Dreams

For a summer in the mid-eighties, I lived in a suburb of Washington, D.C. One night I dreamed that I was working in a Kinko's copy shop, in a high-ceilinged basement of an old building.

The photocopying machines were churning out documents. I was perspiring. The room was miserably hot, the machines endlessly clacked and whirred, and the windowless walls allowed neither fresh air nor natural light into our underground cavern.

The boss yelled at me to hurry with an order. I turned to a co-worker, muttering under my breath.

"I *hate* him," I said, gritting my teeth. "This is a sweat shop. He treats us like slaves. Oh, I could *kill* him."

My co-worker motioned me to follow him to a more secluded alcove.

"Are you really angry enough to kill him?"

"Yes!" I said, my cheeks burning.

"Take this information, then," he said, pressing a yellow piece of paper into my hand. "This gives you permission to detonate one nuclear bomb."

I eagerly jammed the paper in my pocket.

"Don't let anyone else see the paper!" he warned. He stared hard at me until I met his eyes. "Do you promise?"

"Yes," I said.

For the rest of the day I fingered that yellow paper as someone might a love letter. I was eager to tear it open and read the contents.

That evening, I turned on the computer and began to enter data, following the printed instructions. I was gleeful, thinking how this would end my misery with the boss.

"I'll show *him* who's powerful," I told myself.

The screen on the computer suddenly turned black. Numbers began flashing on the screen.

"60, 59, 58, 57."

"Oh, my God," I thought, staring at the screen. "This is the final countdown. The bomb is really going to go off."

Horrified, I ran downstairs and into the street. Now, at 1:30 in the morning, all of the surrounding houses were dark, their shades drawn.

"The bomb!" I screamed. "The bomb is going off in less than a minute!"

No lights blinked in the gape-eyed windows. I was sobbing, alone, in the darkened street.

I ran back to the computer. 10, 9, 8 – the numbers flashed white against the black screen.

7, 6, 5, 4.

My heart was racing. Would the world really end? I closed my eyes and wrapped my arms around my knees.

3, 2, 1.

I braced myself for the heat, for the intense mushroom cloud of light.

The computer whirred and spit out a red paper about the size of a movie-theater ticket. I stared at the ticket for a long time, my breath ragged, with sweat pouring down my back. I realized that the ticket could be used at any time to detonate a real bomb. The computer was a dry run; I had "earned" the ability to deploy an actual nuclear warhead. After several minutes, I reached for the stub and placed it in my pocket.

The next day at work, I looked at my co-workers, wondering if they knew my secret. Could they see or sense the power I harbored in my pocket?

I suddenly had new respect for the President. He had a similar power, the ability to deploy nuclear warheads at any moment. Unlike me, though, the President had a much larger arsenal at his command. And also unlike me, the President had not allowed his personal vendettas to influence his use of the nuclear bombs.

I fingered the ticket in my pocket again. I had a talisman to remind me of my own anger and lust for power. I took a deep breath. I can relax now, I thought. I was in better hands than I had realized. Those national leaders whom I had so deeply criticized had more control than I did.

I awoke from the dream in my sodden bed, with the muggy

night air pressed close around me. That night I felt another piece of my terror about nuclear war slip away. I knew the threat of nuclear war had not disappeared. The new revelation was my own part in creating nuclear war. Each of us holds a ticket, the potential for hate and power-lust and war. Fingering that metaphoric ticket, I knew I had that power, and I was choosing not to use it. I was choosing a different route, a journey that steered away from a nuclear nightmare and toward a world at peace. A true choice was possible only because I had the certain knowledge that I was capable of choosing war as well as peace.

Corn God

This morning I awoke, looked out the upstairs window, and peered into a neighbor's backyard pool house. Puzzled, I suddenly realized I had never seen the inside before because its door was now missing, dispersed in the night's ferocious storm and winds.

The sunflowers in the vegetable garden were a tangled mess. The tallest, most glorious of the sunflowers, standing over 13-feet-tall, had snapped in the gale. Corn stalks were askew, like broken chairs turned upside down. A garden trellis, waiting to be secured in the lawn, was draped over the picnic table. A ficus houseplant, outside for the summer, lay on its side, its terra-cotta pot cracked in half.

As I walked through the neighborhood I saw that the streets were littered with leaves and twisted branches. One woman stood dazed on her lawn, looking at two downed limbs.

"Did we have a storm last night?" she asked.

I nodded.

"I didn't feel well last night, so I guess I just slept through it." She pulled at a limb for a moment and looked up at the tree. "I'll have to call someone to help."

Many neighbors were outside raking leaves, sweeping debris into piles and dragging branches to add to them.

I looked at the tufts of green leaves scattered on the ground and thought of this turning of the season, Lughnasadh, the cross-quarter day in the Celtic calendar between the summer solstice and the autumn equinox. In Celtic tradition, August 1st is a sacred holiday, a celebration of the beginning of the harvest. In this ancient cycle, the Corn God Lugh reaches his peak of power at the summer solstice; then, he is sacrificed on Lughnasadh, cut at the knees, the chest, the throat, pierced with a blade just as the grain stalks are cut with the scythe. That curved blade harvests wheat and rye, corn and millet at this very beginning of the turning of the seasons.

As the Corn God declines, the Goddess gains in strength. With the dying of the summer light, the deep restorative power of darkness begins to accrue. Every August an unexplainable melancholy rises in me as the evenings grow shorter and the autumn flowers begin to bloom.

I tip-toe amongst the tangle of cucumber, watermelon and pumpkin vines in the garden, ecstatic to discover the first red tomatoes, purple bell peppers and smooth-skinned cucumbers. I heft the cucumber in my hand then look out at the downed leaves and branches in the yard. Corn God, I think, severed from the vine at the peak of his strength. The ferocious winds cut these trees at the peak of their summer glory. Even amidst the excitement of gathering first fruits from the garden, I taste a hint of sadness.

Eating cucumber salad for lunch, I recognize that I take others' life so that mine may go on. The wheel of life is exacting; no life continues without some loss to another. I can't stop the turning of that wheel. I can, however, ride as close as possible to the center, minimizing my impact on surrounding life. Riding at the very center, I know my life is inseparable from the whole. I am seed, cucumber, human, compost. I eat myself and am consumed by myself in return. In the center, God and Goddess are one, and I am their progeny.

The Ribbon Demonstration

Justine Merritt, a devout Catholic, believed her life mission was to help bring about world peace by serving as a missionary in South and Central America. She was ready to quit her job and move to South America but wanted to check her inner promptings, first.

"In February 1982," writes Justine, "I went on retreat to pray for guidance for my life. I had been traveling and writing for a couple of years, but something seemed out of focus. I prayed, I realized later, with a divided heart: half of my heart was very earnestly imploring the Lord to guide me, and the other half of my heart was saying, 'and make sure you send me to South America' where I thought I wanted to go.

"But something happened. One morning, again in prayer, the poem 'Gift' was given to me, and even the stubborn, frightened child in me could understand that the path I was to follow led not to South America, but toward working for peace at home."

Justine saw that piece work – an American folk term for needlework and quilting – could become an expression of peace work. A couple of weeks after her vigil, a vision emerged of encircling the Pentagon on the fortieth anniversary of Hiroshima with a ribbon made of many sections, created by individuals and groups to depict what they could not bear to lose in a nuclear war.

She wrote down the vision and sent it to everyone on her Christmas card list. During the next two years, her vision was passed through mimeographed posters, letters, and word-of-mouth until by August 6, 1985 enough people had responded to her vision to circle the Pentagon and stretch an additional *fifteen miles* to include the Washington Monument and the Lincoln Memorial. The three-foot-by-one-foot banners came from people all over the world, expressing what humans love about this planet. Many of the banners depicted the planet Earth, children, forests, air, water and music. Some banners had papers pinned on them that told of the despair the creator had endured coming to terms with nuclear war, and the power that had come from choosing life.

On that muggy summer afternoon, while waiting for the final

link-up of the chain at 2 p.m., I chatted with friends from Connecticut who had ridden all night on a bus to join the demonstration. I walked behind a group of woman-identified spiritualists, their arms linked as they sang joyous songs. They joined brown-robed Franciscan monks who were quietly viewing the banners. Housewives from Iowa were talking about their year-long project of creating a banner together.

"Where is your banner?" I asked. "Is it the one you're holding?"

"Oh, no," said the woman. "I came here to help hold someone else's vision."

At 1:50 p.m. we moved into a line along the four-lane highway just north of the Pentagon. Passing cars slowed, and the drivers honked and waved. A man riding a bicycle stopped in front of me. He looked dazed. I stepped forward and touched his arm. "Are you OK?" I asked.

"It just got to me," he said, his voice cracking with emotion. "I've ridden around all fifteen miles of the banner route and just there, at that corner back there, it got to me."

I reached out and hugged him while he cried. After a couple of minutes, he stepped back on his bike and continued on, tears still streaming.

Two p.m. Balloons rose from the Pentagon lawn. I half expected a thunderclap or a sudden rain shower to bless the moment, but only a low rumble of cheering along the line marked the moment of linkage.

I was familiar with the unexpected welling of tears at a friend's wedding, when two people announced their love for one another, but I had never experienced a community declaration of love.

Acts of love are powerful, even irresistible. An act of love draws people – all people – together, in a way that anger never will.

Today, on another anniversary of Hiroshima, I ask myself again, "What do I adore? What could I not bear to lose in a nuclear war? How can I enact that love in the world, right now, and make my life an expression of that love?"

Playing for Joy

I began playing the violin when I was eight years old. My parents never had to remind me to practice. I played for love of the instrument, and out of wonder at my steadily developing skills.

My last year in high school, I played in the local professional symphony as well as five student orchestras. I really wasn't sure how far my talent would take me, but I knew a music-performance degree would be difficult to come back to, so I decided to begin my college years majoring in music.

Jens Ellerman, my private violin professor at the University of Cincinnati, College Conservatory of Music, was German, and a perfectionist. Once in a lesson I played an entire Mozart concerto. At the end, Jens shook his head in disgust.

"Judith, you made two mistakes. Do you know what they were?"

I nodded my head. "I missed a shift at the beginning of the second movement, and one note was out of tune in the third movement." I hadn't dropped the violin or wet the carpet, but Jens viewed these other minor misdemeanors as felonies.

Jens nodded his head. "Play again, and don't make any mistakes."

I took a deep breath, and my accompanist and I plunged into another 20 minutes of music. At the end, Jens was even more frustrated.

"Judith, you made two *new* mistakes."

I continued to progress over the next year and a half, but not fast enough for Jens. During my last lesson before Thanksgiving break in my sophomore year, Jens stopped me in the middle of an etude.

"Judith," he said in his clipped German accent, "you are so intelligent in other ways. Why can't you be intelligent on the violin?"

His words were carefully chosen and delivered; he obviously had prepared this speech.

"You know, lots of people in this school couldn't do anything else if they lost a finger or were hurt. But you can. So why don't you go do something else?"

Reverend Earl Copes was outside in the hallway during Jens' fateful lecture, waiting to drive me home for the Thanksgiving holiday. Reverend Copes was the minister of music in the church I grew up in and one of my beloved mentors. He was a gifted organist as well as a composer, arranger and conductor. His son, Ronald Copes, is a renowned violinist.

"You know, Judith," he told me warmly as we drove north along the darkened highway, "there's room for people with all levels of ability in the music world."

Reverend Copes had the grace to find healing words to soothe my flayed ego. At the time, I felt he was handing me a booby prize, solid confirmation of my musical ineptness. Now I realize he was offering an avenue for redemption – searching through the ashes of my dreams to find my own gift in the musical world.

I transferred to Oberlin, where I could pursue both music and academics. After graduation, I spent four years living and working outside the United States. When I returned to the States, I lived an hour north of New York City, and I often made trips into Manhattan. One rainy December afternoon I was passing through the waiting room in Grand Central Station when I heard Irish folk tunes played on a hammered dulcimer.

In Grand Central sound seems to blossom from the center of the ceiling. I looked around and finally discovered the source of the music – a man with a scraggly beard and long red hair hunched over a hammered dulcimer. He had a pile of cassette tapes for sale in front of him and wicker basket marked "Tips."

I stopped to chat and mentioned that I had played many of the same tunes in a Ceilidh band in Scotland.

Bill's eyes lit up. "Then why don't you come join me?" he asked. "You could play with me for a day or two the next time I'm in the city."

For the next six months I took the train a couple of times a month to join Bill. We played in Grand Central Station, Penn Station, and the Times Square subway.

We played mostly O'Carolan tunes. O'Carolan, a blind Irish

harpist from the late 1700s, married the heart of Irish folk music with the emerging Baroque tradition. These elegant tunes would roll along the vaulted ceilings of Grand Central, bathing the commuters with simple, heartfelt music. More than one harried commuter would stop to listen and then burst into tears.

"I've never heard music like that," said one man, dabbing his eyes with a cotton handkerchief. "What is it?" In that hard, glitzy city, I realized people were starved for simple beauty.

I also came to know the street people who made the subways their home. Some of them would stop to chat when we took breaks between tunes. At Grand Central Station, an African American man in a wheelchair often stopped to listen. One morning I saw him trying to push open the door to the men's room. No one else seemed to notice him struggling. He looked up and caught my eye as I dodged through the crowd with my violin case tucked under my arm. In that wordless meeting of eyes, I knew he desperately needed to get to a toilet. My first impulse was to push him through the door. I hesitated, wondering if I would start a riot, a woman pushing a disabled man into the men's toilet. I glanced up at the clock, saw that I was late, and grimaced. I met his eyes again, shrugged my shoulders, and smiled. He smiled back.

Ten minutes later, as Bill and I began to play, my friend rolled up next to me and put on his handbrake.

"I come to hear some pretty music," he said.

At that moment I realized the music we were playing had the power to touch people's hearts, to speak in ways that words could not. Although that man and I had never shared many words, he knew me through the music. He knew me through the genius of a blind harper who had died several centuries before. He knew me through the violin-maker who had carved my instrument a hundred years before. He knew me through the love I brought to the instrument and the music, and the way we had learned to sing together. He sensed the love that had traveled through all of those hands – composer, instrument maker, musician – into his heart.

I had begun to play all those years before out of love, and I had allowed my conservatory experience to blight that passion. Now I was playing with the knowledge that this simple, heartfelt music had the power to heal. There in the subways, among my street friends, I had finally found my place in the musical world. I had learned to play for joy.

True North

Soon after I graduated from college, I returned to my high school to visit Mr. Smith, one of my favorite, and toughest, teachers.

After regaling him with stories of college and my time at the Bear Tribe, a community founded by Sun Bear, an Anishnabe teacher, I asked him my pet question of that era:

"Are you happy?"

He looked at me blankly. "Am I happy?" he repeated.

"Yes. Are you happy in your life?"

I phrased the question carefully. I was not interested whether someone was happy *with* their life; I was interested if they were happy *in* it. I assumed that happiness was a compass that pointed accurately toward the true north of someone's destiny.

Mr. Schenk foundered for several moments. "I don't know how to answer that question."

He paused. "You know I've been raising my brother's son, don't you?"

I nodded. I'd heard a few comments while in school, but never knew the details of how Mr. Schenk had ended up parenting his brother's child.

He sighed deeply. For the first time ever I saw his shoulders sag.

"I love Danny with all my heart. He's truly my reason for living. And I never imagined how much work would be involved with raising a child."

My omnipotent mentor, the hard-driving honors-English teacher whom we secretly called "God Almighty Smith," or GAS for short, was suddenly so plainly human, so vulnerable, so windblown by the gales of life.

"How did you end up raising him?" I asked.

"Oh, phew," said Mr. Smith, rolling his eyes. "I was raising my brother after my parents' death. Spring break of his senior year, my brother went off to Florida and got a girl pregnant."

"His girlfriend?"

"No, some girl – excuse me, *young woman* – who was also on

vacation. Anyway, she was willing to have the baby if someone else raised it. So, I said I would raise the child."

He shrugged his shoulders.

"And is your brother helping?"

"Are you kidding?" said Mr. Smith, laughing. "He's still a child himself. Danny's my boy. There's no doubt about that."

I thought back to my junior year when I was studying English Lit with Mr. Smith, and how our intrepid teacher had likely been juggling baby-sitters, diaper changes and bottle feedings while grading our term papers. Today he was no longer masked as my invincible teacher. I saw his vulnerability. I also had a full-frontal view of his integrity.

Mr. Smith definitely seemed to be on course, but happiness was not the only wind filling his sail. I sensed a bone-deep weariness, a breath of resentment toward his brother, and a gale-force love that propelled his life-ship. Following one's deepest convictions, saying "yes" to the unexpected, and enacting one's love did not necessarily add up to happiness.

A few years ago I was talking with a mentor, bemoaning my circumstances as a single working mother. "I just wish I had things a little bit easier. Just a wee bit."

She erupted in a belly laugh. "You think you came here for *easy*?" she asked as she gasped for breath.

I had to laugh, too. I'd been taken with the New-Age notion that being spiritual and being aligned with my life path meant that I would be healthy, happy, wealthy and wise. If I was having a difficult passage, my life must not be on course.

Perhaps some people really do come into this life for an easy ride. I know very few of them. I'm not talking about martyrdom, intentionally seeking out the painful or the impossible. Not many need to seek inclement weather. Most of us encounter hurricanes without having courted them.

Emotions may not be the best compass for finding true north. Emotions color the landscape of our lives, but they are not the substance of our experience. As spiritual teacher Adyashanti suggests, being awake means fully meeting pain as well as bliss. Being fully awake is different from trying to improve the experience of sleep-walking. Most spiritually oriented self-help practices teach how to manifest more money, more love and more stuff. Those practices help create a more comfortable dream. They don't wake me up to the truth of here and now.

Mr. Smith chose with awareness, and he chose with integrity. Being fully awake in his choices did not guarantee an easy, happy life. He did, however, learn to navigate with acceptance, and even joy. In raising his nephew, I believe Mr. Smith found true north.

What's My Line(age)

I am daughter of Martha, daughter of Gladys, daughter of Celeste, daughter of Minerva. These women are the biological river that flows through me, the unbroken cord of my ancestors.

I have explored the ancestral lands of my forebears, walking the cornfields of central Ohio, where the golden evening light of early September hangs like a living blanket on the burnished fields. I have trod through the cloud-shrouded moors of Scotland, and hiked the rolling, stone-studded fields of England. I have sought a sense of home in these far-flung lands, but each time have departed as I had arrived – a foreigner on native soil.

For most of my life I have felt like the swan dropped into the duckling's nest, an alien in what seemed to be familiar territory. When my mother and I go out for lunch, the waitress asks if we want separate checks. We don't argue at the table; we simply bear no resemblance to one another. In fact, I do not look like any of my grandmother's other 12 grandchildren.

Biology does not necessarily rule inner evolution, any more than genes can guarantee physical appearance. I grew up in Ohio but never felt at home there, despite more than six generations of ancestors who had sent deep taproots into the black, fertile soil.

In my late twenties, after I had lived and worked with native people around the world, my mother sent me a newspaper clipping about the Shawnee Nation United Remnant Band buying land in Ohio. I had grown up being told in history class that the Shawnee of Ohio had long since moved west or died of smallpox. What a welcome revelation that native people still lived there.

I wrote an article about the Shawnee for *Cultural Survival* magazine, and returned to Ohio the following spring for the Shawnee Bread Dance ceremony. At the end of the weekend I was packing my car, preparing to join my parents in the suburbs south of Dayton. I was devastated to be leaving the simple gathering of tents, the ceremonial Great House covered with freshly leaved boughs, and the pond with bull frogs chorusing in the late-spring heat of southern Ohio.

"Where are you going?" asked Kiji, the tribe's medicine

person.

"Home to my parents' house," I answered, wiping tears from my cheeks. "But *this* feels like home, right here. I've never felt at home in Ohio before."

Kiji laughed softly and wrapped me in his enormous arms. "This is your home now. You are always welcome here."

And so I began an association with the Shawandasse, as they call themselves, that has continued for almost thirty years. I have felt more at home at Shawandasse council meetings and ceremony than I ever have with my biological family. Lawogway, the sub chief, always invited me to stay with his family when I traveled to Ohio. Perhaps he thought my parents had abused or abandoned me; nothing could be further from the truth. My parents raised me with great love and unwavering support. I have failed in my efforts to explain to him, or even to myself, why I have never found a deep sense of home amidst my closest genetic kin.

Kiji, my Shawandasse mentor, describes with conviction how physical biology determines cultural, social and spiritual orientation, not just eye or hair color.

"Then why do I feel so at home among the Shawandasse?" I asked.

"Well, your family has been here for many generations. Maybe some of them knew and respected Shawnee people."

I sat perplexed, absorbing his words. Gradually I've come to realize I have a very different understanding. Rather than creating elaborate physical explanations for a deep sense of kinship, I recognize that each of us carries one or more spiritual lineages that may or may not match our biological inheritance.

By "spiritual lineage" I mean something much deeper than church affiliation. I'm referring to the deepest roots of spiritual direction, an allegiance that goes far beyond denominations, or even religious lines.

I envy those whose physical, cultural and spiritual lineages are so neatly braided into one smooth, unbroken cord. My own mismatched lineages make a lumpy but sturdy mesh.

"Why wasn't I born in Tibet?" I commiserated with one of my

mentors.

"It's not needed there," she replied simply. "You probably would have been more comfortable growing up on a reservation, or in an African-American community. But you most likely would not have had the strength to overcome the physical challenges and the poverty to do what you are doing today."

Perhaps I chose my biological lineage – white, northern-European mongrel – to serve my spiritual lineage. I sense there are many primary people's souls enfolded in peach-colored flesh. This is not a wishful "wanna-be" stance, hoping to snatch the soul (which is about all that has been left unsullied) of native peoples. No, this is the revelation of a biologically cross-dressed soul. My cover does not necessarily match the contents of the book. If you would know me, or anyone, open the pages and read the tracings of the soul.

I have a friend, born in Harlem, whose father marched with Malcolm X in the early Sixties. My friend feels most at home in the cathedrals of Europe. I know an English doctor who for years dreamed of her Lakota family. I have a mentor, born in North America of northern-European heritage, who is a Tibetan spiritual lineage holder.

Biology is not destiny, particularly where the soul is concerned. We shape-shift in and out of physical envelopes that are appropriate for that segment of our journey. Look within, not without, for the artful braiding of physical, cultural and spiritual lineages that anchors us to our deepest home.

Inner and Outer Technology

The sun blazed in Australia's Gibson Desert as the young girls tugged at my hands, pulling me across the red sand desert.

"Look over here!" one of them called, pointing excitedly. "See those lizard tracks?"

I thought of myself as a fairly astute observer of the Earth, but I had to admit I could not discern the lizard tracks among the rocks and windswept sand. These aboriginal girls, raised in this desert, with a river of 40,000 years of ancestral knowledge coursing through their veins, knew that land in a way I could only dream of.

David, a documentary filmmaker and I had arrived in the western desert a week earlier to record a film about the Martujarra people's struggles with uranium-mining companies moving into their presumably protected lands. We had driven along dirt tracks 1,000 kilometers into the Gibson Desert. The morning after our arrival, officials from a mining company flew into the camp. They wanted the Martujarra people to identify sacred sites so they could avoid desecrating those areas in their explorations.

Hours after our arrival, David and I boarded a plane along with five of the aboriginal men and several mining camp officials to fly even deeper into the heart of the western desert.

After landing, David and the aboriginal men boarded a helicopter, to begin aerial reconnaissance of sacred sites. I was instructed to drive with the cook to the mining officials' camp, to help make dinner. Clearly a woman's place in this male-dominated mining world was in the kitchen. I made some biscuits with self-rising flour and cooked them on the outdoor grill. After tasting the smoke-laced doughy lumps, no one asked me to cook again.

The aboriginal men and David returned shortly before nightfall. David's eyes were alight, describing the desert they had explored by helicopter.

"And then the pilot got lost," said David, his eyes twinkling.

"How did you get back?" I asked, knowing that from the air the desert is a rippling sea of red sand waves, undulating without interruption for thousands of miles.

"Mugi, one of the men, told him the way."

"Mugi? How could Mugi know? He's never been in a plane or helicopter in his life!"

David smiled. "The song lines. Remember? He's known the song lines since he was a small child. He didn't leave the desert until he was six or seven years old."

Thirty years earlier, a few of the Martujarra had left for the cities of northwestern Australia, hoping to better their lives. Instead of physical ease and wealth, however, they ended up in cardboard shanty towns, living on the outer fringes of the city.

The family and community ties that bind the Martujarra were so strong that soon aunts and uncles, cousins and grandparents followed those song lines to the edges of the city. They, too, settled into the shanty towns. Uprooted from the land that had sustained them for so many millennia, the Martujarra became steeped with a sense of hopelessness.

Brian Kelly, an Australian Viet Nam veteran, began to spend time with these aboriginal people. After his service as a Green Beret, mainstream Australian life made little sense to Brian. He found a haven among the Martujarra. For years he listened to the people talk of their homelands and their longing to return. Brian worked with them to write grants that would allow them to return to the desert with some technology to ease their daily life in a fierce desert climate that could freeze at night and rise to 160 degrees Fahrenheit by mid-day.

After several decades of living in the city, and *no* experience of seeing the landscape from the air, Mugi still knew his precise location from the song lines he had learned as a child. These "lines" are the literal trails the aboriginal people walked as they moved from camp to camp across the desert. The songs told of the physical as well as spiritual geography of the landscape; they wove dreamtime ancestral ramblings with morality and practical advice. A song line might begin,

That boulder over there is where Lizard Man lay hiding, waiting to steal food from Snake Woman when she came over those hills. And that mountain range over there, shaped like Lizard's curled tail, is where she

threw Lizard Man when she discovered his plan.

"And that rock where he was hiding, he dropped onion seeds into the ground. Good bush tucker there, wild onions.

"So see, he was really greedy. If he was just patient, he could have had a whole belly full of bush tucker, but instead of waiting and sharing, he tried to ambush Snake Woman. What that get him? Killed!"

So in this story, my spur-of-the-moment example to illustrate a song line, we have physical geography – this rock, that mountain range; we have morality – be patient, be respectful, and share; and we have practical advice – right there, next to that rock, you will find wild onions.

Knowing the desert in such a deep and multi-faceted way, no wonder Mugi had recognized the Dreamtime territory from the air.

Outwardly, aboriginal culture is primitive. When Europeans arrived, the aboriginal people truly lived at a stone-age level of technological development. Their inner technology, however, as demonstrated by Mugi's knowledge of the desert, outstrips almost anything we know or understand in the western world.

Outer technology bends the world to suit us; inner technology reframes the body and soul to accommodate the environment. Outer technologies rely on fossil fuel and other non-renewable resources; inner technologies rely on the strength and ingenuity of spirit.

In the West we have pursued outer technology, developing ever more complicated gadgetry to control the external world. Most indigenous cultures have taken an opposite approach, cultivating their non-physical, inner abilities. In the Martujarra's case, this supreme mastery of their inner world has allowed them to survive more than 40,000 years in one of the planet's most extreme landscapes. The Dreamtime, primitive in outer technology, is much more mysterious, and likely much more sustainable, than the illusory control of Western technology.

Messenger Owls

In the towering elm outside my bedroom window, two owls hooted in the first glimmer of daylight. They chorused back and forth, their throaty baritone notes fluttering down from the leafy branches outside the widow. Song birds screeched and dive-bombed the chorusing pair. Finally, they drifted on silent wings to a neighboring tree, sang another sleepy duet, and then settled into silence.

Many native people consider owl an omen of death. I think of my father, newly diagnosed with a recurrence of cancer, as I consider these nocturnal messengers arriving in the dawn. Are they reminding me that death is a cross-over point, just as dawn links day and night?

I'm wary, waiting for the phone to ring. I also know that this harbinger of death may signal my own demise – the destruction of internal patterns of resistance, fear and frustration. Can I die to others' opinions of me? Can I let go of fear of lack? Can I surrender my financial struggles? Can I lay down the burdens of my life and settle peacefully into this moment, the stillness of dawning light?

Among the Shawnee, owl links the people with their ancestors, creates a bridge to those who have passed before them. What would the ancient ones have to say to me now? What would they teach me about living in transitional times?

My ancestors survived the Black Death of the Middle Ages in Europe and the dazzling, light-filled awakening of the Renaissance. One thread of my family lineage sailed to Plymouth Rock and set foot on a world newly discovered, so foreign to the well-worn land of Europe. Listening to my ancestors I would hear whispers of invasions, cataclysms, revolutions, awakenings – the cacophony of their voices melding into a symphony of hope.

May I be that owlish presence, singing the sun above the horizon as I pass into solar slumber. Waking and sleeping; arising and dying, the quiet fluttering of souls in the tree of life.

Mary Oliver, a poet of awakened heart, offers her own owlish description of mortality.

White Owl Flies Into and Out of the Field

Coming down
out of the freezing sky
with its depths of light,
like an angel,
or a buddha with wings,
it was beautiful
and accurate,
striking the snow and whatever was there
with a force that left the imprint
of the tips of its wings —
five feet apart — and the grabbing
thrust of its feet,
and the indentation of what had been running
through the white valleys
of the snow —

and then it rose, gracefully,
and flew back to the frozen marshes,
to lurk there,
like a little lighthouse,
in the blue shadows —
so I thought:
maybe death
isn't darkness, after all,
but so much light
wrapping itself around us —

as soft as feathers —
that we are instantly weary
of looking, and looking, and shut our eyes,
not without amazement,

and let ourselves be carried,
as through the translucence of mica,
to the river
that is without the least dapple or shadow —
that is nothing but light — scalding, aortal light —
in which we are washed and washed
out of our bones.

Yes, may I pass out of this life and into the next adventure with
my eyes wide open, with light streaming in and through me. May I
follow that radiance to the Source of All Things.

Now, in my waking world, may I ride that luminous ocean
in a coracle of awakening, alert to the light's presence, even in the
maelstrom of shifting darkness. May I focus on that river until the
blaze seeps into my eyes, an ongoing cataract of joy, flowing onward,
onward into the ocean of light.

Poem from: *Owls and Other Fantasies* by Mary Oliver,
Published by Beacon Press, Boston
Copyright © 2003 by Mary Oliver
Reprinted by permission of The Charlotte Sheedy Literary
Agency Inc.

AUTUMN

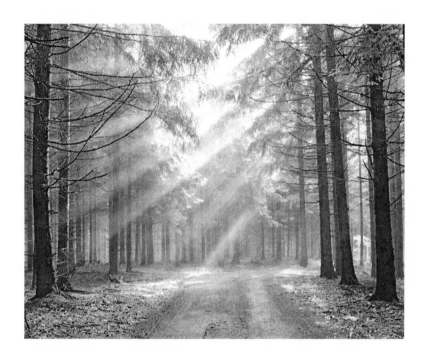

Crossroads

On the autumn equinox after graduating from college, my parents and I traveled to Britain. For three weeks we explored England. I planned to travel alone for another three months, in Britain and throughout Europe, before returning to the U.S.

The first two weeks of my solo journey, I backpacked in England's Lake District. The late October skies turned gun-barrel grey, and rain blew in slanted curtains. The huts and bed-and-breakfasts where I stayed had no central heating. Soon I had a cough, and then bronchitis.

One evening I perused *Let's Go Britain*, hoping to find an inexpensive place to rest for a few days. The most promising was a Tibetan Buddhist Monastery in Scotland called Sam-E Ling. The guide promised three hot meals a day and simple dormitory-style housing for a modest fee. I called and made reservations for a week.

The monastery was an old Scottish estate, the elegant main building built of hewn sandstone blocks. I walked into the main hallway where sweeping stairways curved to the upper floors. One of the staff members escorted me to the second floor and into the dormitory room. 20 twin mattresses neatly lined two walls. Large windows on the far side of the room framed a view of rain-sodden fields and bare-limbed larch trees.

"The dining room is on the left of the entrance hall," she explained, "and the meditation hall is on the right."

"Do you have set meditation times?" I asked.

"Tonight is different," she said. "There's a special ceremony with one of the visiting lamas. You are welcome to come and sit quietly in the back. There are special teachings this week, so the meditation hall will not be open to guests."

That evening I walked into the meditation hall as the ceremony began. A maroon-robed monk with a shaved head handed me a book with a transcription of the ceremony. I settled cross-legged on a cushion at the back of the room and glanced at the book.

I assumed the unfamiliar symbols, with their delicate waves and trailing flourishes, were Sanskrit, the language of Tibet. The monks near the front of the room were chanting rhythmically, following the lines.

Trying to grasp the details, I felt I had landed on the moon. Instead I closed the book and shut my eyes, allowing the rhythm and sounds to transport me to another world. Over an hour passed before the sounds faded, and the ceremony ended.

During the days that followed, I worked in the kitchen, went for walks, and meditated. The morning of my departure, I ate breakfast and then packed my few possessions. I laced heavy boots and hoisted the pack on my back.

As I walked down the curving staircase, I saw one of the shorn nuns at the bottom of the steps. She locked eyes with me as I descended. Her smooth, peaceful face was ageless.

"Where are you going?" she asked.

I laughed, thinking the answer obvious. "To the train station."

"Why are you going?" she asked, her brow creasing.

"Well, I made reservations through this morning . . . ."

"You should say here." Her voice was quiet but firm. "You are very beautiful. You should stay here."

"But I've made plans to go to Findhorn . . . "

"You are very beautiful. You should stay *here*," she repeated.

I paused on the bottom step. I did not realize at the time that she probably recognized me from other lives shared in spiritual community. I also did not recognize her as an embodiment of Kali, keeper of the crossroads, the one who mediates the forked byways in our life passage.

I wish now that I had taken more time at that life juncture to consider carefully the two diverging roads. One led into deep, solitary spiritual pursuit, within the Tibetan Buddhist tradition, a path so familiar on my soul's journey. The other path also led me deeper into spirituality, but within a more socially oriented community.

Both paths beckoned me on my spiritual journey, but with radically different emphases. I chose the less familiar path, a spiritual community focused on group interaction and planetary change.

And in truth, perhaps I allowed momentum alone to carry me. With plans already in motion, I didn't have the sense to stop and reconsider them.

Gradually I've learned to spend more time – sometimes months – at life junctures, waiting with varying degrees of patience for clarity about my life direction.

I wonder sometimes if some part of my soul continues along the road not taken, living out another possible world in some parallel universe.

Like Robert Frost, meeting his fate in a snowy wood on a darkening afternoon, I've almost always taken the less familiar road, the one less trodden, and that has made all the difference since.

Light on the Land

Spring begins cold, storms wet and wild, and mellows into cherry blossoms. Summer runs feral with lazy, hazy heat. Autumn is light, illuminated amber, reflected in an angle of prayer.

I have autumn days stored like holograms in my memory. I remember walking home from school in seventh grade, abandoning the school bus to make the three-mile walk home because I couldn't bear any separation from the crystalline light. The air was absolutely still with the faintest hint of coolness after the inferno of Ohio summer. I walked along the streets that rolled between suburban homes, all familiar territory – I had watched these houses rise like wooden mushrooms from the muddy Ohio farmland. On this day, though, the light transformed all that was ordinary into something beyond physical. Each object stood out, like a cut-out in a story book, in more than three dimensions. When I got home, I still could not walk indoors. I wandered in the garden and gazed at the tomatoes, shimmering ruby red on frosted vines. The lingering calendula flowers stood like yellow suns, their backs arched to catch every dazzling ray.

I chafed against the inward turning of autumn, the forced encampment of school with its dusty books and stained carpet. I welcomed the cooler nights but mourned the early passage of dusk into night.

As an adult, I still feel a pang of sadness, an unnamable grief as the days shorten and the nights cool. I watch two crows wheeling in the sky, cawing conversationally. Are they capturing the last hints of summer in their languid movements and their friendly conversation, before the hard-edged days of winter?

Years ago my parents met me in September at the airport in Columbus. We stopped to eat at the Red Brick Tavern on Highway 40, the National Road, a few miles from my ancestors' homes. After dinner, I stepped into the humid evening air, warm with late-summer sun, and stood transfixed, gazing into a cornfield. The sun, almost level with the horizon, shot gold through the pollen hanging in the motionless air. The illuminated pollen glistened and spiraled, a tiny galaxy of living stars crowning the tassels.

Another autumn I stood on a wooden deck at Hocking Hills State Park. Again the evening air was motionless and saturated with a golden peace. For nearly an hour I stood motionless as tree-fringed narrow valleys slowly filled with shadows, and the sun slipped behind the rim of the world.

The quality of light in those moments literally illuminated some deeper experience of the land, exposing its ephemeral beauty and deeply rooted peace. Always I have been strongly affected by light and have been privileged to experience the angle of light at different seasons on many parts of the planet. I could not explain with a physicist's acumen the reasons why, but I can say without hesitation that the most spectacular autumn light I have ever witnessed was in Ohio.

The stillness was not stagnancy, but rather a held breath, a knife-edged moment of balance. These moments of equilibrium are evanescent, dispersed in the first puff of wind or slowly exhaled breath.

Balance is the ephemeral equality of light and dark that marks the autumn equinox. In truth. this Earth is always losing and gaining, accruing and spending, giving and receiving. Light pours into darkness, losing itself and then threading through the darkest center into light once again. Forever these mates, light and dark, have been waltzing around the wheel of the year. Today, for a moment, they take a breath and pause, celebrating the autumnal light on the land.

Fact or Fiction

In her late fifties, Gail had straight black hair, angular hips, large feet and uneven teeth.

"When I was in my twenties," she said, looking wistful, "I had a figure like this." She traced a perfect hourglass, with curvaceous breasts and hips and a hopelessly small waist.

"People used to stop on the streets to look at me." She nodded with satisfaction. "I was really something!"

Both of us sporadically attended Vipassana meditation class on Sunday evenings. One autumn evening we drove together to class. After "hellos" and comments about the rainy weather, Gail turned to face me.

"I've been writing," she said earnestly. "My autobiography."

"That's great!" I said. I'm always enthusiastic about someone's creative endeavors.

"Well, it's not so great. I realized today it was all fiction."

I stifled a laugh. Her face communicated that she was dead serious.

"How do you mean?" I asked. "Why is it fiction?"

"Oh, like my relationship with my mother. I realized I had made up a lot of – well, stuff. Like what she thought about me, and why she said and did the things she did. And none of it's true."

Later in the evening, during the open-comment and question time, Gail recounted her revelation to the class. More than a hundred meditators burst into gales of laughter. The hilarity, though, was not so much mocking as stunned revelation. How accurately have I recounted my own life, even to myself? How many stories have I fabricated about other people's thoughts and actions, which have in turn shaped my own worldview?

Recently a patient offered another profound angle on personal history.

"I don't have a past," she said simply. "Not really. I have *memories* of my past, and memories of having those memories. But I really don't *have* those experiences, here and now.

Her revelation caught me off-guard. How disturbing and

simultaneously freeing to be orphaned from my past. I realized how comforting those recollections were – even the "bad" or "negative" ones. I can dust and fondle them, like keepsakes on a mantle. Who would I be if I collected them all and left them on the doorstep of a thrift store? What if I had no mental heirlooms to dust?

In clinical hypnosis training, I experienced how the subconscious mind makes a perfect record of all past events, complete with sight, smell, sound, touch and taste. In deep hypnosis, a form of deep relaxation, I have access to that pristine recording of past events.

I believe that record must also lie within our neural tissues. I remember years ago watching a movie of an open-brain surgery, with the neural surgeon touching different parts of the brain to elicit vivid memories from the conscious patient.

"Oh," she exclaimed, "I haven't heard that song since I was in high school!" She sang along with the memory, perfectly recalling every word.

This imprint lies within the physical, neural tissue, the "hardware" of the body. The conscious mind, though, seems to filter these memories, bending them according to its current conditioning.

When I awaken, will that memory-bending prism become a clear, flat glass? Or better yet, will perception enter my awareness with no filtration at all?

For now, I am left only with the present moment – the sound of wind chimes in the restless October winds; the dull ache in my upper neck. Light filtering through the surging branches, and leaf shadows dancing on the carpeted floor. Now silence, as the wind dies. Crickets thrumming – the last who have survived the hard September frost.

Memory creeps into presence. Crickets dying in the first hard frost – that is recollection. I am gathering the tatters of the past. In present moment, crickets sing – nothing more, nothing less.

The past shapes my present. My history grinds the lens through which I perceive the present moment, and my perceptions in *this moment* focus my future.

Here, now, in this moment, I have the opportunity, if I can seize it, to polish the lens, perhaps even *remove* that filter, for a moment of pure seeing.

"If he could teach me to see," says Annie Dillard, "I would stumble across a thousand deserts after any lunatic at all."

Filters transform memory into fiction. Removing those prisms allows me to see reality, to enter the realm of non-fiction. So this art of seeing purely is more about shedding, releasing, discarding – not adding to the picture, but rather meeting it unedited.

Here, now, is the meeting of past and future. This tenuous intersection is the only moment I truly have. Let me hold it with curiosity, with wonder, with generous attentiveness. Without wakeful presence, I will make a fiction of my life.

Until Death Do Us Part

I met Audrey on a Greyhound bus, heading north from New York City. The day before, on a blistering Saturday in early June, we had both joined a million other people in the Peace March, winding through the streets of Manhattan to a final gathering in Central Park. Now, with the demonstration a joyous memory, I was traveling north to my job as a camp counselor, and Audrey was headed home.

I was 20 years old, a mostly grown tree full of sap and newly furled ideals. Audrey was in her 60s, deeply rooted in her family, and branching into new interests of her own. She had recently returned to college to finish an undergraduate degree in women's studies.

As we began to share our lives and hearts and ideas, a spark flared and then caught between us. We were ripe for revolution. The many entwining branches of our lives ignited like dry tinder in that unexpected blaze of minds and hearts. During that three-hour journey, before she stepped off the bus in upstate New York, that spark flared into a roaring blaze that endured for the rest of our lives.

That summer I kept up a steady correspondence with Audrey. We wrote more sporadically through the rest of my college years, and then during my travels abroad. We wrote of our families, our passions and our desires for the world. We wrote about the things we loved, and the sorrows that etched their own patterns on our hearts.

When I graduated from medical school, Audrey enlisted her daughter, who lived in a neighboring city, to take me out to lunch. Then in her 70s, Audrey was traveling less frequently and apologized for not making the 3,000-mile journey to the graduation ceremony. I delighted in her daughter Victoria's company. I also marveled at the strength of this connection with Audrey, then more than a decade strong, ignited by a three-hour bus ride, and since nurtured only by letters.

Our correspondence lapsed for a couple of years. I knew that Audrey had moved, as my holiday letters came back stamped with "No forwarding address." Soon after I began working for a company that made women's health supplements, the receptionist handed me a letter with a familiar, artistic scrawl. I whooped with delight as I read the return address – Audrey. She had been surfing the company's website when she discovered my name among the list of physicians.

"I just knew it had to be you!" she wrote. "I've moved, and wanted you to have my new address."

Soon after the boys were born, Audrey called from the retirement home where she and her husband had moved. I delighted in hearing her voice, for the first time in almost twenty years. Audrey, my long-time friend, was just as close as ever, yet I also sensed her slipping from me physically as her life force began to dim.

A few years later, Audrey's holiday greeting was brief but poignant. Her husband had died, and she was ready to follow. "Don't worry, I'm not suicidal," she wrote. "I still have my family, my beloved children and grandchildren. But I deeply miss my husband."

This January, Audrey's holiday letter came back again, stamped with "No Forwarding Address." I spent an hour trying to find her on the internet. I tried several phone numbers, without success.

A couple of weeks ago, Audrey's daughter, Victoria, left a message on my voicemail, asking me to call. That night, as I worked with my son to put fresh sheets on his bed, a picture cube embedded with my parents' message to the boys spontaneously began to play. The message played through twice, ending with, "We love you very much."

"Hmmmm," said Sebastian. "That's weird. No one pressed the button."

When I called Victoria the next day, I was not surprised by the news that Audrey had recently passed. We shared stories and laughed and cried about the richness of Audrey's life. Amidst my tears, I celebrated the passion with which Audrey had lived, to have touched my life, and so many others, so deeply.

And I realized that Audrey had already come to say good-bye in her own way, tripping the voices on the picture cube. "I love you, too, Audrey," I said out loud after hanging up the phone. "I love you, too."

Length of contact does not dictate depth of love. Knowing Audrey was like stepping into a stream of love and conversation that had no beginning and no end. I knew her, I know her, and I will know her. All are true. All are different aspects of the same stream. I trust our paths will cross again, on some unexpected byway down the road.

The Last Time

The last time I turned the lock on my house in Portland, my home for nine years, the door shut behind me with a heavy thud. The gates swung closed on an entire era of my life. I stood on the wooden porch, knowing I could not re-enter. I had already checked each room twice. The air was thick, moist and expectant. I knew what I was leaving, but I was uncertain about what I was entering.

The last time I saw my fiancé, my first great love, he had curly hair and a closely cropped beard. His yellow shirt blazed against summer-brown skin. I knew the taste of his full lips, the softly toned elasticity of his skin, and the musical rhythm of his love-making. Our lips met, lingering, and our hands trailed to our sides. I watched him step onto the train, and caught his brave smile as he half-turned to wave.

My last day at Findhorn in Scotland, I moved half-dazed around my bedroom, picking up old letters, half-read books and mismatched socks. The last ten percent of any packing seems to be the hardest: those lingering items never had a permanent home, and that indigent status makes them even more difficult to command in the final organizing. At last, the room emptied, I vacuumed and then closed the latch, one last time.

My father is preparing to travel to Nebraska, to see the family farm and walk upon the upturned earth, jubilant with towering corn. One more time he will walk those rows and talk to the farmer about crop prices and fertilizers, pounds per acre and machinery.

For six months I worked in a nursing home and witnessed so many last moments: the last fresh peach to pass through Mabel's eager lips; the final letter Sylvia dictated to her granddaughter, with the promise of Hanukah Gelt; the last view of scarlet and amber maple leaves before the wind and rain scoured them from the branches.

The last time. How lucky I am when I can swing a gate shut behind me, with full awareness of the finality of my action. No lingering, messy endings. No slowly dying wounded beast. Let me end full stop, at the apex of my strength.

So many endings come unplanned: the unexpected death, the

rogue storm, the freak accident. Those endings leave a trail of detritus: the words never spoken, the photos never framed, the letters never answered.

In my grief, in the weighing of those final moments, let me add joy to the measure. May I find joy in savoring the last cherry of the season, the final leaves of basil before frost blackens them, the last lingering kiss.

Learning to pass through these gateways with complete awareness, with my raw heart fully unfurled, I'm practicing for the final release – my own passing from this world. Sogyol Rinpoche explains that Tibetan Buddhists practice dying, not out of morbidity, but rather out of a desire to *live* fully and completely. Rather than being distracted by volunteer work or family demands or cross-stitch samplers, the elders of the Tibetan Buddhist community spend much of their final years in meditation, preparing for their passage from this life. From their perspective, the more peaceful and joyful their exit from this world, the more auspicious their next incarnation will be. In other words, the way they leave this life is a springboard for the next.

I've grown used to emotional whiplash, the soul-snapping rebound I endure trying to clutch at desired objects as the river of life pulls me relentlessly forward. Slowly I'm learning to let go before the rapids wrench those beloveds from my arms. What if I could leave all of those coveted states of being on the bank, before even entering the river? What if I could live with open hands and open heart? What if I could practice dying so fully that I was eternally alive in this moment?

The last time I draw a breath, may I let it go with ease. Like Gandhi, may I have Creator's name on my lips. May I go shining, joyfully closing the gate behind me, and opening my heart to all that lies before me.

Healing Stones

Brad arrived at the Findhorn Foundation during the second autumn of my stay there. He was a guest, I was preparing for membership, and both of us were cooking lunch that week in the kitchen.

Brad shared with the group early in the week about his poor eyesight. He had had numerous surgeries for brain cancer, some of which had affected his vision. On his "up" days, he could laugh and joke about his "hard head," the occipital shell that had been fashioned out of the same material as dentures to replace the skull bone that had been eaten away by cancer. Some mornings, though, he looked gray, and the effort of standing seemed to overwhelm him.

On one of his stormy mornings, I asked Brad if I could give him a healing treatment during lunch. I wanted to support him and, in truth, I also wanted to assuage my own pain. My beloved Aunt Muffy had died of cancer eight years earlier. My mother and I were leaving to be with her when the hospital called to say that Muffy had died alone, lying on a dirty bedpan. I was offering my support not only for Brad, but also for Muffy, and for anyone else who was alone, in pain, or dying.

Brad humored me. We walked up to the healing sanctuary and he rested on the table while I laid my hands on his head, chest and back. After a silent hour, he rushed out of the room to catch a bus to another part of the community.

Later that week during our morning sharing before work in the kitchen, Brad wrestled with the idea of "unconditional love."

"I know my kids love me, but I don't think anyone else *really* loves me. Not without expecting something back."

No one commented. One of the hallmarks of such sharings at Findhorn is "no cross-talk." The speaker has the circle's full attention. That person's truth, in that moment, stands unsullied, unchallenged.

The following week, the community hosted its autumn conference, an international gathering focused on spiritual practice. Brad and I exchanged a few "hellos." He looked relaxed and peaceful.

At the end of the conference, I saw Brad across the auditorium. He was wearing a business suit, and his face looked stony.

"I have something for you, Brad," I told him as I gave him a hug goodbye. I pressed a stone into his hand, a flat, round stone worn smooth in the tides of the North Sea. "This is to help you remember that there really is such a thing as unconditional love."

"Thanks," he murmured as he stuffed the stone in his pocket. He gathered his coat and walked swiftly from the auditorium.

Eighteen months passed. I was supervising clean up after dinner when Brad burst through the kitchen door.

He was beaming as he pressed the beach stone into my hand.

"I've been carrying this since I left the community," he said. The stone had a new sheen, polished by sweat and constant handling. "I want to give it back to you, and boy, do I have a story for you.

"I never really had time to tell you about what happened when you gave me that healing treatment. When I was diagnosed with brain cancer, I let myself feel the terror for about 20 minutes. Then, I cut off *all* feeling. I never allowed myself to even consider dying. I became a guinea peg. I would go to Grand Rounds at the hospital where I worked, and the students would stare at me like a monkey in a cage.

"Well, when I was lying on that table, I experienced my death. I let myself feel the terror, the pain, the sadness. I lifted out of my body, my head bobbing up like a monstrous balloon, and I died right there on the table."

Brad's eyes sparkled. "When I left here and went back to the United States, I had another CT scan and they found a new brain tumor. I decided this time I was going to be *grateful*. I really heard what Brother David Steindl-Rast said in that conference, that gratitude opens the door for miracles. So I decided that no matter what happened I would be grateful.

"I was in the hospital the night before surgery, and the nurses kept commenting on how peaceful I was. After the surgery, when I woke up, I kept focusing on gratitude. I felt so much better than after any other surgery.

"And then the surgeon came in and told me that he had been able to completely remove the new tumor. It had been growing in just the right place to cut off the blood supply to a couple of tumors at the back of the brain that had been there for years, that couldn't be removed without killing me. Those inoperable tumors had died, and the surgeon was able to remove the debris."

Brad's eyes filled with tears. "For the first time in ten years, I have no cancer in my body."

He gave me a bear hug.

"You are a miracle," I told him, tears streaming down my face.

If stones could talk, this one would sing of gratitude, of death squarely faced, of life lived like treasure gleaned from a full-moon tide. If you were here, I would press this stone into your hand, and tell you that love is real, and that gratitude opens the door to miracles.

A Mystic's Halloween

When I was five years old, I wore the family hand-me-down Halloween costume. I was an Indian, complete with turkey feather head-dress and a fringed brown cotton tunic. I danced and warbled a war cry for the neighbors, held out my pillow case, and then sat grinning at the kitchen table with my booty of apples, Tootsie Rolls, and candy bars.

Soon after I outgrew the Indian outfit, my parents had no money for store-bought costumes, and my mom was too busy to sew one. Most years I stuffed a pillow inside one of my father's worn woolen shirts, jammed an old stocking cap on my head, and blackened my face with charcoal.

"What are you?" asked one of the neighbors, eyeing me quizzically.

"A hobo," I said definitively. "Can't you tell?"

Now when my boys whine and beg to go to a box store to buy a costume, I smile. "How about being a hobo?"

"A *hobo*?" they repeat, incredulous. "What's a hobo?"

"You know, someone who rides the railways and lives in the woods."

"But I want to be a vampire!" says Sebastian. "I'm tired of being a ninja."

"How about a hobo vampire?" chimes in Jeff.

The boys start to giggle.

"How about a hobo vampire teen-age mutant ninja turtle?"

Now the boys are rolling in the back seat.

"How about," says Vincent, gasping, "a hobo vampire teenage mutant ninja turtle super hero?"

This playful banter reminded me of one of the deeper meanings hidden in the Halloween celebration. When Europeans first arrived in North America, they were surprised to discover that several native nations already had a similar celebration among their people. On October 31st, they took on new roles – cross-dressing, wearing animal skins, adopting the habits and manners of others for the day.

In Celtic tradition Halloween, or Samhain, marked the end of the old year, when the veils between this and other worlds were the thinnest. The ancient Celts understood that this time was ripe for honoring and contacting their ancestors. The Catholic Church capitalized on this aspect of the holiday by naming November 1st, the beginning of the new year, "All Saints Day." Many traditional Catholics still clean and decorate their ancestors' graves on this day and pray for their passage into heaven.

The other aspect of the holiday *not* adopted by the Church was the understanding that our character and habits are malleable. Stereotyped, culturally mandated roles could be parodied or shed, and new skins adopted – for the day. At this cross-over point of the year, I can cast off what is no longer needed and experiment with new forms.

Will I play with beauty – the princess archetype – or with power – super heroes and politicians? Will I dabble with fearful monsters, vampires, or zombies?

I can don or drop these robes as I please, shape-shifting in and out of new forms in a culture rich with structures to hold me in a particular mold.

On Halloween, those cultural norms collapse, in preparation for the passage into a new year, and the possibility of new ways of being.

As our human society careens toward a time of massive restructuring, perhaps I can use this holiday as a practice for the coming era. I'm not invoking apocalypse, but rather experimenting with robes and skins befitting a new understanding of the Earth and our human role in its evolution.

Perhaps I'll fashion a costume of the Crone, mediating at the crossroads of choice and transformation. Maybe I'll adopt the garb of evolutionary artist, brushing with pure light instead of paints. Perhaps I will be energy healer, needing only my mind, heart and hands to make myself and others whole.

What costume will you wear this year? Don't be surprised if you open the door and find a cosmic vampire hobo ninja mystic healer on the doorstep. Please be kind and fill my bag with treats of the holiest kind: relics of saints, gems and pearls, dreams and inspired visions. I can't wait to count my booty at the kitchen table.

Autumn Leaves

Yesterday in the garden, the temperature peaking at 45 degrees, I was entranced with the Bradford pear leaves, falling meteors of translucent orange, gold and scarlet. I would prop the shovel in the freshly turned garden dirt and wander to a newly fallen leaf to marvel at a circle of gold etched on scarlet, at the way the light illuminated another leaf so that the smooth surface seemed to glow from within. I made some progress in the garden, but more importantly, I fed my soul autumn color and light.

I've been homesick for the mountains in Colorado, more this season than any other. What has filled my heart here, though, in the northeastern corner of Oklahoma, is the festival of leaves and birdsong.

In October, during a restless, sleepless night, I heard an owl in the backyard for the first time since moving here. I had heard the call of an owl at dusk in a distant part of the neighborhood, but never had I heard the velvety hooting of an owl at such close range in our new home. I lay and listened through that unending night and finally rose early in the morning to walk. About a mile from home, along a street lined with oaks, an owl – my owl? – swooped down, in broad daylight, about six feet from my shoulder.

My walks this autumn are often interrupted. I spy an oak leaf, burnished burnt amber with five perfect limbs. I tuck it in my pocket. A cottonwood leaf, liquid gold at the edge of the road, catches my eye. I have discovered more than six species of oak, each shedding a distinctive leaf. These treasures, too, I have carried home and slipped between the pages of books. Almost every thick book in the house has at least a dozen leaves pressed between the pages. I'm completely taken with the plethora of shapes and colors and textures among the leaves.

Some evenings the wind is restless, and so am I. I sit at the computer, watch a YouTube video, read a chapter of *Writing Down the Bones*, look for a paper I've misplaced, and then finally I settle in the chair with a pen, close my eyes, and listen to the wind surging like an unseen river across the land.

So much of this land is shaped by this relentless, invisible force. Leaves pile up below the front-porch step and congregate in the corners. The uninhabited rocking chair creaks in the gusts. Walking yesterday, I watched a pile of leaves lift from the curb and circle, like a ring of fairies dancing, until the wind gently dropped them to the street.

Like the wind-driven leaves I, too, am moved by invisible forces. I dress in the morning, choose my breakfast, drive through the dawn-burnished streets. I think I'm in control, watching other cars stream by, observing thoughts flow like dust motes through my mind.

In control of *what*? I ask myself. Am I really in control? And is control something I ultimately want?

Chogyal Rinpoche speaks of compassion arising naturally, spontaneously. Compassion is self-arising, like a flower that unfurls because it must, not because it has to. Compassion arises like the fairy circle of leaves, a spontaneous eddy in this ceaseless movement of wind.

Who would I be, *what* would I be, if I let go of trying to be good? Would I gorge myself on a gallon ice cream? No, I think, feeling slightly nauseated at the thought. Would I leave my children, run away from my job, abandon my partner, rob a bank?

I sigh, then laugh. No, I think, shaking my head. That's not in my nature.

Nature often is used to connote all that is not human. Here, though, nature points to what is innately human, meaning what is uncontrived, unmolded, relaxed, at ease, just itself. Nothing added and nothing subtracted. Simple.

Unsettled, swirling, arising, settling. My thoughts and feelings, the leaves on the curb – all are moved by the same wind. Just as the wind surges and eddies, howls and sighs, so does all that is innate in me rise and blossom, fade and fall, taking a form that wholly suits itself.

Dancing in the Penitentiary

During the autumn of my fourth year in medical school, I received a letter from an inmate in a minimum-security prison in Washington state asking for help in organizing a pow-wow. A regional coordinator for a Native-American community had forwarded the letter. She attached a moderately coercive note reminding me of my debt to native people and the legacy of our now-deceased spiritual mentor, an Anishnabe elder named Sun Bear.

I remembered that one of my classmates had volunteered with Native-American inmates in the Oregon prisons. She gave me the name of the Lakota Club at the Oregon State Penitentiary, or OSP, and suggested I call them. Maybe someone there could coach me in how to organize a pow-wow in prison.

I called and left a message on the answering machine for the Lakota Club. An inmate named Gary returned my call, saying he would be happy to provide information about setting up a pow-wow. He invited me to come for the next pow-wow, scheduled for a month later.

"We just need your name, date of birth, social-security number and address," said Gary.

"What for?" I asked.

"To put you on the visiting list," explained Gary. "They'll run a background check on you. They have to do that for everyone who comes in here. I'm sure you'll have no problem."

During the next month I tried desperately to find someone to go with me to the pow-wow. No one was available. My options exhausted, I resigned myself to driving alone to Salem, over an hour's drive to the south, to face the prison on my own.

Sodden leaves carpeted the walkway leading from the parking lot to the prison entrance. I walked carefully, aware of watchful eyes from the gun tower in front of me.

I walked past the yellow brick guard tower and up the stairs into the waiting area. A round desk sat squarely in the center of the room. Lockers lined one wall and cushioned metal chairs stood at attention in neat rows in front of the desk. I approached the desk and stood in line behind a family waiting to sign in.

"Name?" said the guard. "Driver's license or other identification?"

I fished in my backpack for my license. He took a long time finding my name, a last-minute addition at the bottom of the list.

"I also brought these for the Lakota Club," I told the guard, opening a paper bag filled with tobacco, sage and a braid of sweet grass. In a traditional culture, visitors always bring gifts. I wanted to bring something useful, so I chose herbs that have spiritual significance in Native-American culture.

"You can't bring those in," said the guard.

"Oh," I said, "aren't they allowed to use these in ceremony?"

"You can leave them here," he said, nodding his head toward the desk.

"And you will give them to the Club?"

"Look," said the guard, "we have to check everything that comes into this place. We used to allow people to bring food into the pow-wows, and then someone brought in marijuana cookies. Ruined it for everyone. Now we can't allow any food, or anything else that hasn't been checked."

I smiled wanly, then shuffled across the room to deposit my coat. I sat shivering, a cold draft slicing through the window cracked open behind me.

After everyone had signed in, we waited to be called forward, in groups of five. To pass through the metal detector, we stripped all metal from our body.

We moved through a series of gates and metal doors. The guards in "command central" checked our ID's a second time. Finally we moved down a long hallway, our moccasins scuffing the well-waxed floor. We moved in single file through the last door and into the visiting room.

I breathed deeply. Sound enveloped me, drumbeats pressing into my body. Two inmates, wearing jeans stamped with "OSP" and pow-wow ribbon shirts, greeted me. I scrawled my name in the guest book and then moved into the linoleum-tiled visiting room, where more vinyl-covered chairs were arranged in rows. In the far corner, a group of inmates were drumming and singing, the sound booming in this hard-shelled room.

One of the inmates stood and invited guests dressed in regalia to join the Grand Entry. Two elders I had seen greeting each other near the front desk stepped forward, along with several other outside visitors, and a few inmates who were dressed in full dance regalia.

I watched the procession of elders and dancers, standing as they passed, and then waited with bent head as Martin Eder, the leader of the Lakota Club at OSP, offered a prayer. He made a special prayer for the inmates on death row, the ". . . brothers who are waiting . . . for justice." The inmates rumbled in quiet agreement, scuffing their feet, nodding heads.

As I watched the dancers moving toe-sole, toe-sole in a rhythmic two-step, one of the guards approached me.

"Here," he said smiling, holding out the packet of herbs that I had left at the front desk. "You can give this to anyone you want."

"Thanks," I said, nodding.

The music stopped, and a give-away began. I edged around the room to where Martin Eder sat, a worn drum-beater resting on his lap. I crouched beside him and gently touched his arm. He turned toward me, patient, quiet. His face was cocoa brown, the color of prairie grass in winter, and thin, black, hair hung below his shoulders. His scraggly beard was shaved into a goatee.

"I brought these for the Club," I explained, handing him the bundle.

He nodded slightly, dipping his eyes. "Thank you," he murmured. He looked up, our eyes meeting. We smiled at each other.

An honor song followed, to acknowledge Glenda Durham, a lawyer who was investigating "chemical restraints," or over-medication of native inmates. Glenda stepped forward, wearing black tights and a big button-down shirt, her beaded moccasins treading lightly on the polished floor.

As the dances continued, I began to sense the good feeling and reverence that infused the space. As I gazed around at the inmates, men of all ages, races and body types, I saw them more clearly as

people. Take away the denim pants with their red "OSP" mark, or
the black lace shoes, and they could be waiters, cooks, salespeople,
accountants, neighbors . . . . even friends. They could be human
beings living in cages, and their captors, fixated on their captivity,
mistaking them for animals.

I drove back to Portland in silence. I breathed deeply, grateful
for the relative freedom of my life, and the privileges I take for
granted each day.

I also marveled at the love that bloomed in that hard-edged
place, despite all of the restrictions, rules and attempts to bar contact.
Spirit seeped into that place, shape-shifting between bars and steel and
reinforced glass. Creator was alive among the inmates, the costumed
dancers, the visitors, the orange-coated guards. I expected fear and
violence to greet me, and instead was welcomed with love.

Heart Talk

Very few people from the town of Forres ventured anywhere near the Findhorn Foundation in Scotland. Among the locals we were known as "hippies." The Home Office named us "harmless eccentrics." Other than guests who joined me in weeding, planting, and turning compost, I had few interactions in the rambling one-acre vegetable garden.

One day a man in neat tweed trousers and jacket strode into the garden. He paused to lean on his walking stick as he eyed the ripening strawberries.

"Hello!" I called, looking up from the kale bed.

He smiled and walked over to join me.

"I'm Jimmy," he said, extending a hand.

I shook his hand. "Pleased to meet you, Jimmy. I'm Judith."

Over the next six months, Jimmy became an increasingly frequent visitor in the garden. He would stroll through the beds, poking at weeds with his walking stick and making friendly chatter. He'd bring seeds or cuttings from his garden, tucked into his tweed jacket, and remind me when I needed to seed or prune something.

Over time I discovered Jimmy, retired and in his early 70s, made a daily 20-mile loop, walking through the town and surrounding countryside.

"My cousin was working at one of the estates, repairing something in the main house," recalled Jimmy, a twinkle in his eye. "He asked if I wanted to come along. I was sitting at the kitchen table, talking and laughing with a woman. She got up to make tea. My cousin came round the corner and said, 'You know who that is?'

"I shrugged my shoulders.

"'That's lady so-and-so. You shouldna be talking with her so common-like.'

"'We're just talking. Any harm in that? She's a human being, just like me.'"

The longer I lived in Scotland, the more radical I understood Jimmy to be. In his quiet way, with his elven mischief, he was breaking walls of etiquette that had been built over millennia. The

class system carefully separated the lairds from their servants and
sharecroppers – how else could they justify this radically unequal
distribution of wealth, work and power? The concept of manifest
destiny – one to rule, the other to live under the foot of the master –
had been practiced for centuries.

Jimmy had either missed that history lesson or he had chosen
to ignore it.

Over time I began to sense Jimmy's secret for how he had
come to mingle with such a diverse clan, including the likes of me.
One day, I was weeding a bed of snap beans, struggling to bury my
disappointment over a performance I was preparing with three other
Foundation members.

Jimmy appeared in the garden, a ready smile on his face. He
balanced his hands carefully on his cane and squared his feet.

"All right then, Judith. What's bothering you?"

I looked up and forced myself to smile. "I'm fine, Jimmy.
Nothing's wrong."

Jimmy shook his head. "A problem shared is a problem halved.
Now tell me what's bothering you."

Tears scalded my cheeks. I spilled out my struggles with the
mutinous actors.

Jimmy didn't ask questions or offer advice. He knelt down on
one knee and placed his arm around my shoulder.

"There," he said simply. "A problem shared is a problem halved.
Are you feeling better?"

I gave Jimmy a sodden hug. "Yes, I do. Thanks, Jimmy."

When Jimmy knew I was leaving the Foundation the following
January, we extended our talks and lingered longer in "our garden,"
as he called it. On Christmas morning he slipped into Cluny Hill, the
mid-nineteenth century hotel cum community center, to deposit a
tiny box under the tree.

He stood amidst the Foundation members, watching quietly
as I unwrapped my box. Inside the tissue paper I discovered a fine
Irish-linen handkerchief.

I knew instantly who had left the package and wrapped Jimmy
in a bear hug. He tolerated my embrace, straightened a button on

his jacket, and blushed deeply. I knew he was pleased with my response.

Jimmy had never attended a workshop, yet he taught me more about communication than all the experts I've endured since. He had a deeper, more instinctive training – he loved the world, he loved himself, and he found that same love reflected in other people.

His heart talk was as free as his laughter, as unpredictable as the Scottish rains. He had all the trappings of a master – no pretense, even less pride, and an unfathomable well of love.

And Then There Were Three

Last Tuesday, the call came. My father was failing – quickly. My brother had been trying to call me for three days and had left messages at two different phone numbers, but none of the messages had come through. Finally, on Tuesday, I knew my father was close to passing.

The next morning I boarded the plane to Dayton, Ohio. My brother Tom and I talked as he drove me through the back streets, under the steel-grey sky, to the in-patient Hospice Center. Tom shared the many items on my dad's "bucket list" he had helped complete – paying someone to finish and fly a model airplane Dad had been working on for 15 years; sailing a remote-control model sailboat on my brother's pond; attending the Old Timer Model Airplane Competition in Indiana. My dad was not interested in traveling to Paris, or even his birthplace in Toledo, Ohio. He wanted to stay close to home and close to his heart, spending time with his family and flying the model airplanes he had loved since childhood.

When I walked into the hospice room, I was momentarily shocked. Dad's hair, always a lush white flat-top, hung in lank strands around his face. His neck was skeletal, and his mouth a dark, cavernous "o." When he heard my voice, though, he turned and smiled, his sapphire blue eyes dancing with light and life.

We visited for a couple of hours. My dad, brother, mother, two nephews and I were perched amiably in a hodge-podge of chairs. Dad, unable to talk, mouthed words. Some of them I understood. He alternately listened, stared above at the ceiling, and worked restlessly with his hands – turning imaginary screws, smoothing the wood, clearing tools from the invisible work bench.

I stretched out my palm. "Here, Dad, I'll take it." He carefully placed the imaginary screw in my hand. "I got it," I said, placing the invisible tool on the bedside table.

Conversation flowed around the room. "This is like family dinner!" said my nephew Bill. We laughed.

Later that evening, we all went home. I was just stepping out of the shower at 11 p.m. when my mother reported the Hospice nurse had called.

"He's really slipped in the last few hours. She thinks he'll go in the next day or two. Tom is going back to Hospice."

"So am I," I said. "Do you want to come?"

She nodded.

Within an hour we were sitting with Dad, the core of our family. Thirteen years ago, before my sister's sudden passing, we were five. Now, in the darkened hospice room, we were four. As I nestled on the foldout chair-bed, I recalled the last time we had all slept in the same room, nearly 20 years before, in a cabin at family camp in Michigan.

We took turns sitting with Dad or snoozing in the reclining chairs. I was running on three hours of sleep the previous night, and alternated between meditation and a restless doze.

Dad's breath became ragged as his lungs began to fill. The nurse administered more morphine. His breath eased and slowed, eased and slowed, gradually quieting until the tide went out and did not return.

Tom sensed the final moment and reached for Dad's hand. "You can go," he whispered. "It's all right to go."

Fluid came up as his spirit surged upward – moving up, up … free. And then silence.

And then we were three.

We hugged and expressed our love, then sat for an hour with Dad, sharing memories of his life.

At 5:45 a.m. I drove home with my mother. In the pre-dawn darkness I crawled into my childhood bed. Although exhausted, I slept only an hour or two.

When I awoke, I lifted the shade on the second-story window and watched the birds in the crabapple tree. Cardinals, robins, tufted titmice and chickadees were singing and feasting on the frozen apples lingering from last autumn's harvest. They were accruing life from the detritus of the previous season.

My prayer, like the birds: gather nourishment from the passing season. Harvest the elders' stories, celebrate their lives, and make a feast of the living.

Kingly Giving and Receiving

In my early twenties I lived in the Findhorn Foundation, an educational and spiritual center in the north of Scotland. Each December community members gathered to place their names in a hat for a game of "Angels and Mortals." We each secretly drew one name from the hat, and that person became our "Mortal." For the next month, until Christmas Day, each "Angel" was responsible for overseeing the care of our fatefully chosen "Mortal" by anonymously leaving small gifts or arranging special happenings.

One year, I drew my roommate Susan's name from the hat. I began to plan what I would do for her. Knowing she was diabetic, I purchased a sugar-free carob bar and stashed it under her pillow.

When she discovered the carob bar the next morning, she sighed, clearly exasperated.

"My Angel doesn't have a *clue* about what I like," she said.

She missed the momentary hurt that registered on my face. I bit my lip, knowing I could not react to any of her comments without divulging my identity.

"I know what I'll do," said Susan. "My friend Carol wrote a long letter to her Angel with a list of everything she liked and wanted. Carol figured her Angel had no idea who she was or what she liked, because the gifts were so off-base. I think I'll do the same. Then I won't be so frustrated. It should save a lot of hassle for my Angel, too."

Later that day, I received a three-page letter addressed to "Susan's Angel." She carefully outlined what she wanted and noted she hoped the letter would help as "you clearly don't know me very well."

I read the list and began to incorporate what I could. I also created other surprises, like finding someone to read Susan a story in the evening and then tuck her into bed with a cup of hot tea. I created a treasure hunt, complete with mystical clues about the stations on life's journey. The hunt took her to remote parts of the sprawling, nineteenth-century hotel where we lived. The clues brought her back to the same starting place, where a final note read:

We shall not cease from exploration
And the end of all our exploring
Will be to arrive where we started
And know the place for the first time.
        T.S. Eliot, 4 *Quartets*

Susan gave me a detailed description of her treasure hunt that night. "It was so cool!" she exclaimed. "I think I'll set up the same treasure hunt for my Mortal."

For once, I knew I had scored.

Christmas morning arrived. The community buzzed with an extra level of holiday excitement, as this was the day our Angels would be revealed. Each Angel had wrapped one final gift for his or her Mortal and placed it under the tree. The card accompanying the gift was signed with our earthly names.

Someone dressed as Santa began to distribute the gifts. Excited squeals of laughter punctuated the gift opening as Mortals discovered the identity of their Angel.

Susan opened her gift.

"Oh, how wonderful!" she exclaimed as she read the card. She looked across the room and smiled at me. "Thank you!"

I smiled back. "You are so welcome!"

A couple of minutes passed. Susan was standing at my side, her brow creased with concern.

"Judith, did I hurt your feelings with some of the things I said?"

I reached up and gave her a hug.

"No, Susan, not at all. I learned a lot about giving and receiving."

In truth, I *had* learned a lot. In Buddhist teachings, they speak of "princely" and "kingly" giving. When I gift someone, do I extend that present with as much inner wealth and generosity as a prince, or a king? Do I give fully and completely, or am I miserly in my giving, worried about my own loss?

That December I learned an equally great art, that of "princely" and "kingly" *receiving*. Can I receive the gifts offered me with as much grace as a prince or king? Can I receive the love embodied in each gift, regardless of whether I like the object or not? Can I hold that gift with gratitude, as if I held a precious diamond in my hand?

I began to see that I can experience giving only if someone else is able to receive. I can extend the same grace to another person by deeply appreciating the gifts I receive. In a culture that focuses so much on *getting*, we seem to have lost the art of *receiving*. Perhaps Susan, like so many of us, wanted to get the things she wanted more than she wanted to receive what her Angel had to give.

I wonder how many gifts my celestial angels have tried to give me that I have been unwilling or unable to receive? How often have I rejected gifts because they were the wrong color, the wrong material, poorly timed, too expensive, too cheap, too big, too small . . . the list is endless. In the process I realize I have cut myself off from the *love* that was embodied in those packages. I have divorced myself from the grace my angels tried to extend.

"We are each other's angels," a friend recently reminded me. I continue to practice the art of both kingly giving and receiving. I'm far from perfect. I hope I haven't offended my angels too badly with my pauper's skill.

Winter Solstice: Sun Stands Still

The light is fading, and the sky is bending down to bathe the powdery snow with topaz blue. The moon has not yet risen; I'm watching for that light to spread pearlescent over the silent, waiting fields.

Each evening, when the boys are finally quiet, asleep beneath their quilts and blankets, I turn off all the lights except the strand of colored holiday lights framing the back window. I sit alone in the darkness, taking in the silence like soul-nourishing food.

I remember coming home from college for a January term and walking through the darkened streets to a local park surrounded by second-growth forest. Snow crunched beneath my boots on that subzero, windless night. The moon illuminated the open fields, but I sought the shadows of a stand of trees and waited, my breath billowing silver in the moonlight.

The night rewarded my silent watch. I heard an owl hoot in the woods to the north, and another answer from the trees in the east. Their calls volleyed back and forth, a musical exchange of passion during this icy mating season.

I listened for almost half an hour; then, I added my voice to the symphony. We made a trio, the owls and I, hooting across the silent, moonlit field.

I also found that deeply nourishing stillness during the Christmas-Eve service in the church I attended throughout my childhood. Returning home to visit my parents on Christmas Eve, I sat in the familiar polished maple pew and smiled with delight as I recognized the rich symbolism I had grown up with, now appreciated more deeply with an accumulation of diverse cultural and spiritual experiences.

A magnificent pine tree towered to the left of the altar, decorated simply with white ornaments, Christian symbols that adorned a much older icon – the evergreen tree, the one that never dies in winter's most bitter grip, the life that survives the deepest inward pull.

I felt my own Celtic roots tingling, the older European traditions that had melded with Christianity as it surged north from Jerusalem and flowed even into the Irish villages of my ancestors. Christ permeated those older roots, spreading golden light among the craggy roots of the tree of life.

I followed responsive readings, quietly changing the patriarchal language to suit my own truths. I remembered the alto line of the carols without opening the hymnal.

And then my favorite moment of the service arrived. The lights dimmed to total darkness. The minister stood before the only light in the sanctuary, a single candle lit in the Advent wreath.

He lit the other candles on the wreath and then walked down the altar steps to where the choir members stood with their unlit candles. From the darkness, from the solitary flame at the darkest point of the year, the flame passed from hand to hand, from choir members to the people sitting in the pews, the glow traveling from the edges of the sanctuary inward, the light strengthening as people raised and lowered their candles in unison, with the refrains of "Silent Night."

Tears rolled down my cheeks, and the solid alto line faltered. I'm not sure what the other parishioners were celebrating in their hearts, but I knew what was in mine:

Out of the darkness comes the strongest light.

Out of the longest night of the year comes the most potent seed.

I celebrate the return of the sun, the physical light that kindles the world.

I celebrate the rich, deep darkness that nourishes that seed of light.

I honor the point of light within darkness, the seed of yang within the greatest yin.

I honor the owls seeding life at the most inward time of the year. New life springs from the coldest, hardest ground.

I held the candle, with paraffin running over my waiting fingers.

The light is returning. Pass it on.

The light is returning. Tip your candle into my flame.

The light is returning. Pass it on.

We are the seeds of light.

Hear me calling on this moonlit, winter night.
We are the seeds of light.

About the Author

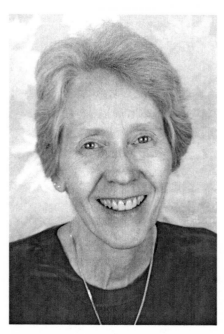

Dr. Judith Boice's spiritual journey began as a teenager backpacking in the Rocky Mountains, Smokey Mountains, and Green Mountains of Vermont. During these explorations of elemental living, she discovered everything around her was alive. This mystical understanding infused all of her life, leading her to live at the Bear Tribe, a Native American Medicine Society founded by Sun Bear, an Anishnabe elder; The Findhorn Foundation in Scotland; Auroville in south India; and with the Martujarra, traditional aboriginal people of Australia's Gibson Desert. This mystical, earth-centered spirituality informed her choice of medical careers. The journey continues now with annual, silent backpacking retreats in the Haleakala Crater on Maui.

As a naturopathic physician and acupuncturist, Dr. Boice focuses on creating health rather than simply eliminating disease. Her concierge practice combines cutting-edge, scientific medical research with the ancient roots of healing practices that address emotional, mental, spiritual as well as physical health. Her work bridges the worlds of science and soul.

Dr. Boice has additional training and experience working with cancer patients and is board certified in naturopathic oncology [Fellow of the American Board of Naturopathic Oncology (FABNO)].

Dr. Boice reaches an international audience through her websites www.greenmedicineacademy.com and www.drjudithboice.com. The Green Medicine Academy offers trainings in green or "classical" medicines, the older systems that predate conventional medicine. Dr. Boice is a regular guest on radio programs and webinars. A member of the National Speaker's Assocation, she is an articulate, inspiring speaker who reaches listeners with a combination of story-telling and technical know-how.

Other Books by Dr. Judith Boice

The Green Medicine Chest: Healthy Treasures for the Whole Family, Morgan James, 2011 (Winner of Nautilus Book Awards Silver Medal and Living Now Book Awards Bronze Medal)

Menopause with Science and Soul: A guidebook for navigating the journey, Ten Speed Press/Celestial Arts, 2007 (Winner of Nautilus Book Awards Silver Medal)

Mother Earth: Through the Eyes of Women Photographers and Writers, Ten Year Anniversary Edition, Sierra Club Books/U.C. Press, 2002 (Winner of Living Now Evergreen Gold Medal, 2014)

"But My Doctor Never Told Me That!": Secrets for Creating Lifelong Health, Althea Press, 1999

The Pocket Guide to Naturopathic Medicine, Crossing Press, 1996

Mother Earth Postcard Book, Sierra Club Books, 1993

Mother Earth: Through the Eyes of Women Photographers and Writers, Sierra Club Books, 1992

The Art of Daily Activism, Wingbow Press, 1992

At One With All Life: A Personal Journey in Gaian Communities, Findhorn Press, 1990

About The Publisher

Lorian Press is a private, for profit business which publishes works approved by the Lorian Association. Current titles can be found on the Lorian website www.lorian.org.

The Lorian Association is a not-for-profit educational organization. Its work is to help people bring the joy, healing, and blessing of their personal spirituality into their everyday lives. This spirituality unfolds out of their unique lives and relationships to Spirit, by whatever name or in whatever form that Spirit is recognized.

For more information, go to www.lorian.org.

CPSIA information can be obtained
at www.ICGtesting.com
Printed in the USA
FFOW02n1409281217
44175542-43577FF